MW00330175

THE WELLNESS ROADMAP

THE
WELLNESS ROADMAP

A STRAIGHTFORWARD GUIDE TO HEALTH AND FITNESS AFTER 40

ALLAN MISNER NASM CPT

Host of The **40+FITNESS** Podcast

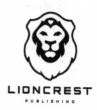

LIONCREST
PUBLISHING

THE WELLNESS ROADMAP
A Straightforward Guide to Health and Fitness After 40

ISBN   978-1-5445-1296-9 *Hardcover*
            978-1-5445-1295-2 *Paperback*
            978-1-5445-1294-5 *Ebook*

This book is dedicated to my wife, Tammy, and our children, Bekah, Cory, Jesse, and Summer. It is the joy they've brought to my life that has made my journey to wellness possible. You are, and will always be, my why.

CONTENTS

DISCLAIMER

I am a personal trainer, not a nutritionist or a doctor. The information I provide in this book is the start of your education, not the end of it. Any tactics or nutrition plans I refer to in this book should be implemented with the guidance or supervision of a medical professional. The following content is based on self-experimentation and testing I've done over the course of years. This is education, not a prescription.

INTRODUCTION

My fat butt sank into the sand of Puerto Vallarta, Mexico, as I meditated, feeling the tide rhythmically rising to meet my feet and falling away again. I had recently purchased a time-share just up the beach, and this was my attempt at taking a vacation.

That moment on the beach was the beginning of a journey for me, and I'm not talking about the plane ride to Mexico. I took that trip down to Puerto Vallarta without knowing exactly where I was going or why—I only knew that I couldn't stay in my comfort zone anymore. I needed to change.

Despite the sound of the waves and the salty smell of the sea breeze, I couldn't bring myself to relax.

How could I? I was just a day short of thirty-nine, and

already I was unfit for my favorite activities. I wanted to meditate in this beautiful environment—I *needed* to meditate—but my thoughts kept drifting back to the day before, when I'd played beach volleyball.

I love playing beach volleyball, and I'd been looking forward to it ever since I'd seen it on the resort's daily activities schedule. I'd arrived early and started playing in earnest, but for the first time in my life, I'd had to sub out of a game—not because I wanted to give someone else a chance to play. I didn't have the energy to keep going.

My own mortality was staring me in the face. I didn't want to be an old man, but here I was, the day before my thirty-ninth birthday, and I couldn't even play volleyball anymore. My work was stressing me out, I was in a toxic relationship, and at that moment, I weighed over 250 pounds (I wasn't sure exactly how much—I'd given up stepping on scales).

As I vacationed in paradise, with palm trees swaying around me and the sun shining each day, every morning I woke up, I felt worse and worse. My waistline had ballooned out, I was drinking heavily, and frankly, I'd turned into a jerk. I thought stress from work had caused my downturn, but I realized in that moment on the beach that it was my health that kept me from enjoying anything. I was fed up with everything I'd become. I used to be an athlete. I used to be in great shape. I used to *like myself.*

What happened?

I opened my eyes from the meditation and looked down at my belly. My stomach hung out over my shorts, and I struggled just to stand up. When I finally did, one of the vendors selling jewelry on the beach happened to pass by with his box. I knew many of the vendors because they played volleyball with us. He'd seen me come out of the game, sweaty and nearly passing out.

"Good morning, Allan. Are you going to play today?"

I shook my head. "I need to ask you a favor, Luis. Can you take my picture?"

He gave me a very confused look, but he took my camera. I knew that if I shied away from this feeling of hopelessness, I would keep returning to this place.

I made him take two photos: one of my front and one of my full-body profile. Nobody would naturally pose for such an unflattering picture, but I wasn't looking for a Facebook profile picture—I wanted a kick in the butt. Nobody looks great from the side unless they've done some serious work to get in shape. I hadn't done the work. I wanted those pictures as a reminder of who I'd become and a solid piece of evidence that this was the worst I'd ever get.

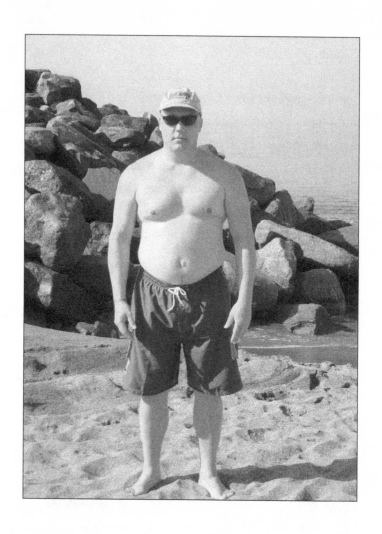

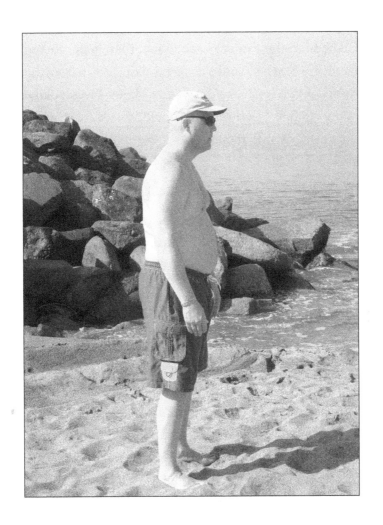

He handed the camera back to me, then kept moving down the beach toward a couple walking down from the resort. When I checked the photos, I knew I was looking at my "before" pictures. My shoulders slouched over a doughy body with mounds of fat like rolling hills on my chest and belly.

This was the moment I would finally change. I would stop being afraid to step on the scale, I'd stop eating horrible food, and I'd cut down on the alcohol. It had been my choices that had turned me into a fat bastard. Now it was my decision to turn my health around—before it was too late.

Maybe it *was* too late.

Whether they want to lose weight, stop smoking, or run a 5K, everybody starts with a decision. But making the decision isn't enough. Decisions are dependent on willpower, a fickle resource. You don't start down the road to wellness with *a decision*—you start with a commitment, and I hadn't made the commitment yet.

Why else would I spend the rest of the week at an all-inclusive resort in Mexico eating and drinking my ass off?

THE WAVES OF RECOVERY

When I got home, I made what I thought were sweeping changes to my life. I eased back on the alcohol, I exercised more, and I cut calories. At first, it worked. I actually lost weight, sometimes as much as fifteen pounds in a month, but inevitably, every time I made progress, the momentum swung the other way, layering the fat back onto my body.

Like the tides of the ocean on that beach in Mexico, my efforts to improve myself came in ebbs and flows.

During one of those cycles, I got down to 230 pounds, which was a huge improvement but still way too heavy for my body. I hadn't addressed any of the underlying issues that sabotaged my health, such as the toxic relationship with my girlfriend at the time and my stressful job as vice president of internal audit for a large corporation. When neither your work life nor your home life offers you any reprieve, you find other ways to cope. For me, it was booze and bad food.

Every time my willpower ran out, I'd find myself in the bottle a little more, and then I'd skip my workout the next morning. Without making an entire lifestyle overhaul, once those surface-level practices of wellness went away, I was back to putting on the weight. I drank alcohol because it relaxed me. I ate garbage fast food because it relaxed me. These coping mechanisms were exactly what my mind thought I needed in the moment, but they were doing awful things to my body.

COMMITMENTS OVER DECISIONS

The reason I kept sabotaging my long-term efforts to get well again was simple, really, when I look back on it. I wasn't practicing self-love. I'd attempted the easy, surface-level changes such as cutting calories and easing back on the booze, but I didn't change anything fundamental about my life, such as my toxic relationship or my stressful job. I relied on pure decisions to make the changes in my life without restructuring everything around myself to support a commitment to health.

This focus on willpower and decisions over true commitment to your goals is the same reason why only 9.2 percent[1] of New Year's resolutions succeed: willpower is a limited resource. If you rely on willpower alone, it will eventually fail you.

Resolution, willpower, decision, and *diet*—we use these words to rationalize failure. They all imply finite terms:

---

1   "New Years Resolution Statistics," Statistic Brain Research Institute, https://www.statisticbrain.com/new-years-resolution-statistics/75.

- Resolutions last for only a year, if you even make it that long.
- Willpower runs out.
- Decisions fade from memory as quickly and as often as you change your mind.
- Diets are something you go on for a finite period of time, which implies you'll eventually go off them.

Commitment, on the other hand, is long term. In a marriage, you commit emotionally to your spouse, now and forever. The same way you commit to a spouse, you must commit to yourself and your wellness.

After that moment on the beach, I rode countless waves of wellness and fatness for eight years, until I eventually found myself lying in a hotel bed, hungover and fat again, still in my toxic relationship and a stressful job, albeit at a different company. I'd put myself through intermittent torture for nearly a decade, but what had it gotten me?

When I sat in Puerto Vallarta in 2005, I'd made a *decision*. In that moment lying on a hotel bed, I finally *committed*.

Then, after years of driving toward my vision, I went from too fat to playing beach volleyball to running a Tough Mudder race with my daughter. But I'm getting ahead of myself—that story is for later. For now, let's cover what you'll learn in this book.

WHAT YOU'LL LEARN IN THIS BOOK

Before I take on a client, I ask them what they want to accomplish and why. I do what's called a root cause analysis: I keep asking "Why?" until I understand what the person is *really* after. Ninety percent of them say they want to lose weight; almost none of them immediately know why.

That's what I'll teach you in this book: how to find your unique *why* for your fitness and wellness journey.

HOW TO FIND YOUR *WHY*

Although I'll use clients, podcast guests, and myself as examples throughout this book, the reason why you want to achieve your wellness goals will be different. In fact, your own *why* can change over time.

I've had clients, for example, who used to derive a lot of enjoyment from playing tennis when they were younger, but now their bodies won't allow them to play. I've had other clients whose body weight is so high they can't complete a hike like they used to. Some people are bedridden, with a doctor telling them if they don't change, they'll die.

Everybody's *why* is going to be different. That's one of the most wonderful parts of life, actually. You could look at the activities you're not able to do anymore—such as tennis and hiking—and feel wistful about what you've lost, but it's part of the beauty of life. We change over time. This book will help you ensure that your changes are for the better and that you can regain the activities you've lost.

HOW TO FIND YOUR VISION

Your vision is what you aim to achieve on your road to wellness. Keep in mind that your vision isn't necessarily the highest possible pinnacle you could reach or the most difficult goal you can imagine—it's the precise image of what you want. Whether you want to run a 5K, do a pull-up, or play tennis on a club team, your vision is what gives you direction.

Your vision might be a feeling, rather than a specific look, and that's normal. As you come to understand what true wellness means for you, you'll gain a greater appreciation of the person you are capable of becoming.

You may encounter switchbacks on the road toward your vision, but those steep roads zigzagging up a mountain are there for a reason: because they help you reach the summit. When you look back on the difficulties on your road to wellness, you'll see that they made you stronger.

Your vision should scare you slightly. You should look

at your vision and say, "I don't know how I'll ever reach that point." But you'll know in your heart that is where you belong.

In this book, I'll teach you how to harness that fear for a better chance of success.

HOW TO CREATE THE RIGHT HABITS

If you were being completely honest with yourself, you'd cut through the excuses and admit that it's not a lack of time keeping you from building the body and lifestyle you want.

You just haven't built the right habits.

The people who wake up every day at 5:00 a.m., with their gym bag already packed and their mind ready to work out, don't do so because of willpower. They've created a habit.

Habits are closely related to commitments, but they're not the same. Here's the key difference: habits are a *result* of the commitments you make. If your spouse needs a ride home from the airport tomorrow at 7:00 p.m., where are you going to be at 7:00 p.m.? If your answer is anything other than "At the airport," then, I don't know about you, but I'd be sleeping on the couch.

You would be at the airport on time because you've made

a habit of taking care of your significant other. Why don't you show that same level of love to yourself?

Building healthy habits is an act of self-love, and the sad truth is that most people don't love themselves as much as they should. If you create the good habits, and work to eliminate the bad ones, you create balance in your life, which allows your body to heal and allows you to travel along your wellness roadmap. That's what I'll teach you in this book: how to build the habits necessary to reach your goals.

HOW TO EDUCATE YOURSELF

You can walk into a bookstore, pick up a random diet book, and read some directive such as, "Don't eat meat, or else," but that doesn't mean you've educated yourself. You have to experiment to find what works for you. We have an infinite amount of information available to us, so separating the wheat from the chaff is a huge challenge, let alone actually implementing the information.

We weren't born with an owner's manual. What works for me may not work for you. You have to get out of your comfort zone and experiment. For these health and fitness experiments, you are the only subject. This is called an "n = 1" experiment. In a health study, the number of participants is represented by n, so if the study has 500 participants, then n = 500. The experts conducting the study then analyze the results, ignoring the outliers (the items that are far outside the range of normal). You don't have 500 of yourself, or outliers—you have only one: you. So every new thing you try will have a tiny, yet incredibly important sample size: you.

I'll help you decide which experiments are worth running and which ones should be left to the mad scientists of the world. I'll also teach you how to educate yourself to create a sustainable lifestyle that fits your unique *why* and *vision.*

ACCOUNTABILITY

If you're married, you probably didn't do the ceremony in secret. Now, there's a chance you eloped, but odds are, you followed a common pattern: you got engaged, you announced the engagement, you had a few parties— bachelor, bachelorette—and then you had the wedding ceremony. You had a constant string of announcements telling the world, "We are making a commitment to each other."

You likely don't put much thought into why, but what you're doing with these announcements is creating accountability. Everything from the rings to your new titles—husband and wife—keeps you accountable to your commitment. Does that mean you'd cheat on your loved one if it weren't for the marriage and wedding ring? Absolutely not! But these actions help reinforce to the world that you're accountable for your relationship.

Once you ride off into the sunset with your new spouse, you don't *automatically* get a "happily ever after" fairytale life together. You work with each other to make adjustments and develop a joint lifestyle. Over the years and decades with your spouse, you both let go of the habits that don't support your shared vision, and you replace what you leave behind with new ones.

Likewise, on the road to wellness you'll eliminate the activities that might cause you to stray, and you'll add more accountability.

A popular quote from motivational speaker Jim Rohn says that you are the average of the five people you spend the most time with. When you were single, you might have gone out with your drinking buddies, but now that you're married, you're accountable to someone else, and you might have to part ways with old company who aren't helping you move toward your vision.

The same way you make more couple friends once you're married, you'll have to find fitness-minded people to support you and keep you accountable on the road to wellness.

If you are truly committed to changing your life, and people who don't want change surround you, you'll encounter some incredible challenges in this process, especially in the beginning.

Your friends might try to hold you back. In this book, I'll teach you the warning signs of potential saboteurs, how to handle them, and how to choose an accountability partner, such as a coach who will help you succeed on your road to wellness.

HOW TO HANDLE SUCCESS

The day will come when you reach your wellness goals. It will be an incredible achievement in your life, but your success will come with its own unique stressors. If you're not the kind of person who's used to being the center of attention, it'll be difficult when people come up to you saying how good you look or that they see you as an inspiration.

It might sound counterintuitive, but I see a lot of clients regress once they reach their goal, *because* of all the positive reinforcement they get. This happens for a few reasons:

- Some see their road to wellness as only a temporary change and therefore aren't fully committed to it.

- Some have external factors out of their control, such as family illness or an accident, that cause a U-turn.
- Subconsciously, they don't feel like they deserve the success or the admiration.

Will you have enough self-love to accept your own success?

As you can imagine, 90 percent of coping with this part of the process—the best part, really—is a mindset shift. I'll teach you how to make that shift.

WHAT THIS BOOK IS AND ISN'T

This is not the weight loss equivalent of a get-rich-quick scheme. Sure, if I really wanted to, I could help you lose seventy pounds in two months. I refuse to take clients who want quick, superficial success, so I certainly won't teach you how to do that here. Empowering my clients is incredibly important to me.

Moreover, weight is only a single data point—and not a particularly good one—that people place far too much significance on. The more important focus of this book is making you happier, healthier, and fitter. When I was sitting on the beach, I wasn't happy, healthy, or fit.

Just as it is harder to remember the planned route when you're the passenger of a car and not the driver, rapid weight loss doesn't teach you how to keep it off. That's why I call this book *The Wellness Roadmap*.

This is not a weight loss book, nor is it a diet book. This is not a training manual that will tell you how to build the perfect abs, or sculpt a lean, athletic body, or be the strongest person at the gym.

This book will not teach you biohacks, all those supplemental shortcuts you can take to improve your body or performance. For most of us, biohacks are a distraction, which, by themselves, don't lead to wellness.

Yes, we will talk about nutrition, and yes, we will go over some training protocols, but more importantly, this book is designed to help you take care of the larger aspects of health and wellness—the elements you need to get under control before you should even *think* about supplements and tricks.

Through a process of self-discovery, self-awareness, and mindset shifts, I will help you create your unique wellness roadmap. The plan that you build throughout this book will not only start you with an excellent foundation, but it'll also drive home the key principles that will help you keep moving forward in your journey, even after you've reached your initial goals.

WHO AM I?

I'm Allan Misner, and I am no longer the fat bastard watching life from the sidelines. On my road to wellness, I became a National Academy of Sports Medicine (NASM) Certified Personal Trainer with specialties in corrective exercise and fitness nutrition. After earning those certifications, I realized that most people over forty need guidance and coaching, so I also added a functional aging specialty from the Functional Aging Institute (FAI).

As I continued to learn, I started the 40+ *Fitness Podcast* and community (40plusfitnesspodcast.com). This podcast and community were predicated on the fact that over 75 percent of Americans are overweight or obese.[2] I want to help reduce that percentage in any way I can.

Initially, my podcast started as a way to record conversations with my clients, just as an easy way to get the message of wellness out to the world. But over time, as the audience has grown, I've refined the show and have interviewed more than 175 health and fitness experts, most of whom have written books—on everything from ketosis to getting stronger to managing hormones.

---

2   Cheryl D. Fryar, Margaret D. Carroll, and Cynthia L. Ogden, "Prevalence of Overweight, Obesity, and Extreme Obesity among Adults Aged 20 and Over: United States, 1960–1962 through 2013–2014," Centers for Disease Control and Prevention, https://www.cdc.gov/nchs/data/hestat/obesity_adult_13_14/obesity_adult_13_14.htm.

I realized something as I trained my clients—both online and offline—and continued the podcast: I was helping people build their wellness roadmap. I was giving folks a true understanding of not only how to get started but also how to learn what works for them and where to go after they reach their initial goals.

The number of people I could help was limited to my clients and podcast listeners, so I decided to write this book as a way to bring my personal training approach to a wider audience.

HOW TO USE THIS BOOK

I've structured this book to reflect the way I coach my clients. It's broken into three parts: GPS, STREETS, and CARGo.

Even though the STREETS section contains most of the actionable advice I use with my clients, I strongly encourage you to go through the GPS section first. You may feel like you're making great time, but if you're driving in the wrong direction, you're not going to be very happy with the results. The GPS will ensure you get where you want to be much faster.

GPS

Before you get on the road to wellness—driving toward a place you've never been before—you have to map your path. Back in the day, before we took a trip, we pulled out the atlas, grabbed a red pen, and drew the route on the map. Nowadays, the GPS does most of the work for us, but we still have to plug in the right coordinates. So in part 1, I'll help you establish your foundation to figure out where you're going on your wellness journey and how to use the most efficient route.

STREETS

Once you've established how you'll reach your destination—or at least the direction you'll start driving—you'll then move into part 2, STREETS. Streets are the conduit to connect your starting position to your final destination, whether those streets are fast-moving, like highways, or slower, like back country roads. In this part of the book, I'll help you develop the strategies and habits to navigate the streets toward wellness at a speed that's right for you.

Not everyone drives a stick shift, some cars require different types of fuel, and some people make more pit stops than others. Likewise, you will need different training regimens, nutrition plans, and rest programs to achieve your goals. That's what we'll cover in part 2.

CARGO

Finally, in part 3, CARGo, you have finally reached your destination. You've gone around roadblocks and construction sites, and you've likely rerouted multiple times, but you finally got to your wellness goal.

Now what?

You look different. People treat you differently. Your entire life—not just your body—may be completely changed. Now might be the time to rest, stop for a beat, and unload your cargo. But your journey doesn't stop there—it's just the beginning. Part 3 will serve as a shorter guidebook—as opposed to a collection of chapters, like the other parts—to help you reset your GPS to your next location and develop strategies to drive forward again.

But there we go again—getting ahead of ourselves. Your journey to your wellness destination can't start until you've set your GPS for the first time.

Are you ready to set your coordinates?

PART 1

GPS

In order to find out where you're going, you must take an honest assessment of where you are. In part 1, I will teach you how to ground yourself in the reality of your health and wellness situation. You'll create your vow to yourself, determine the *real* reason why you want to reach your destination, and learn how to personalize common tools such as SMART goals and baseline health markers to reach your wellness destination.

When you start on the wellness journey for the first time, you'll risk going too hard too fast. Part 1 will help you utilize self-awareness and emotional drive to push yourself down the road without burning out your engine.

CHAPTER 1

GROUNDING

Todd thought he was in the hospital for a bacterial skin infection. He never expected the doctor to tell him he was about to die.

It was 2011, and Todd had just been admitted for cellulitis. The dire seriousness of his situation didn't sink in until Todd's doctor weighed him: the scale read 589 pounds.

The doctors sent him through a battery of tests every day, eventually sending nine different specialists to work on him, all flabbergasted because they'd never seen anyone like him before. Every day they found some new ailment with him. They discovered that he was prediabetic and anemic, and he had arterial tumors on his legs that left puddles of blood whenever he sat.

The doctors were amazed he had walked through the front door of the hospital.

During one of his first days of treatment, Todd lay on his hospital bed as his doctor, two young daughters, and wife of twenty-five years stood in the room with him.

"There's no other way to put this, Todd: if you don't change your lifestyle," the doctor said, "you won't make it five more years."

Todd couldn't believe it. He was in his early forties at the time. He looked over to his daughters, both staring uncomfortably at the cold tile floor, unable to make eye contact with their father. He realized in that moment that if he did die, his daughters wouldn't have any pictures to remember him by. Like most obese people, Todd avoided cameras like the plague. Once you see your weight reflected back to you in the form of a picture, you can't lie to yourself anymore.

Todd had certainly lied to himself. He'd convinced himself he was a victim—that his weight wasn't his fault but rather the result of poor genetics. The rose-colored glasses he wore had blinded him, and it wasn't until the doctors took them off that he could see the truth: the fear in his daughters' eyes.

Todd grounded himself in that moment. He decided that he wouldn't be a victim anymore—he wouldn't wait to be saved. He had to save himself. Upon his release from the hospital, he immediately set out to research the best ways to journey down the road toward wellness.

Todd wasn't concerned with looking good shirtless or bench-pressing 250 pounds. He needed to get healthy so his daughters wouldn't have any more experiences of their nearly 600-pound father lying in a hospital bed or worse.

Todd couldn't exercise due to his myriad of conditions, so he focused all of his attention on his nutrition. Multiple health-care professionals had told him it was impossible to get healthy without exercise: "You can't burn the calories fast enough," they said.

If Todd had listened to the pervasive medical mantras out there, he would have failed.

Instead of focusing on what he *couldn't* do, he recognized his limitations and found ways to work around them. He started a low-carb Paleo nutrition plan and found accountability from a website called MyFitnessPal. He put in the work where he could and let everything else go. Through patience and persistence, he stuck to his plan, and it paid off.

Five years later, he was no longer on his deathbed. He'd lost 323 pounds.

Although losing the equivalent weight of two entire people was a significant mile marker to reach, Todd still had a lot of work to do.

He couldn't have made any progress without taking an honest stock of where he was, grounding himself in reality, and moving forward with a full understanding of his goals in light of his limitations. Rose-colored glasses and all.

I've built out a Wellness GPS Workbook to walk you through all of the steps for setting your GPS. You can access it at wellnessroadmapbook.com/gpsworkbook.

We start with grounding because you need to know where you're going and why you need to be there. I prefer to start with the question "Why?"

EMBRACING YOUR *WHY*

When I spoke to Todd about the moment of change, I could feel the love he had for his daughters, the fear he had about leaving them fatherless, and the pain he felt giving them that terrible memory of him in the hospital bed. He knew getting healthy would be a long trip, but his *why* drives him each and every day.

When considering a long drive—and yes, wellness is a

long trip—you will consider whether the trip is worth the effort and time. I live in Pensacola Beach, Florida. I just plugged Philadelphia into Google Maps, and it shows me that it would take me seventeen hours to drive there. I'd have to have a pretty compelling reason why I'm going, to convince me to make that drive.

NO FLIGHTS AVAILABLE

Before you recommend I get on a plane, I have to inform you that there are no flights to wellness. You have to put in the work to either drive or walk.

Your *why* is going to be the reason you get in the car and keep driving. It will keep you on the road even when times get tough, and it will be a huge part of the joy you'll feel when you get there.

THE CHARACTERISTICS OF A GOOD *WHY* ARE:

1. Deep

2. Emotional

3. Generally fixed

When I'm working with my clients to help them find their *why*, I always bring up self-love, which is critical for making the lifestyle changes necessary for true wellness. Love changes us for the better, and self-love *empowers* us. When we start our wellness journey from a place of self-love, nothing can stop us.

Your wellness *why* should hold just as much emotional weight as your marriage commitment. You should want to show yourself as much love as you showed your spouse when you said, "I do."

Todd's *why* was his wife and daughters. My *why* was my daughter, Bekah. I've since gotten married, so my *why* has changed slightly to include my expanded family. In general, though, your *why* will stay mostly fixed. So when a potential client tells me they want to lose twenty pounds, I know we haven't found their *why*. If they lose that weight, their *why* will go away. That's a formula for yo-yo weight gain.

DO YOU *REALLY* WANT TO LOSE WEIGHT?

Todd was successful because he was emotionally invested in the outcome. He wanted to make damn sure that his daughters saw a healthier daddy before his time was up. He committed to his vision as though he'd married it.

You *must* do the same with your own wellness.

When people come to me saying they want to lose weight, I will press them to find a deeper *why*. This might go on for three or four levels. Quite often, I'll hear, "Because I want to fit into a smaller size dress."

My answer? "If you didn't lose any weight, but you could still fit into and look great in a smaller dress, would you consider that a success?"

Almost invariably, their answer is yes. Most people have never thought about weight loss in those terms before, because up until that point, they'd mistaken the side effect—the lost weight—for their desired result.

Their mistake often leads to failure because they've overlooked the reason why they do *anything*. Todd didn't lose weight because he set out to lose weight: he lost weight as a positive side effect of eating healthier to save his own life and see his daughters grow up.

Weight loss isn't a good *why*, but it is a likely side effect of finding wellness. Dig deep to find a *why* that will sustain you.

HOW TO CREATE A VISION

If you look in the dictionary, it has a very different definition of *vision* than I do. The dictionary says vision is "a thought, concept, or object formed by the imagination." My definition of vision is you living your happiest, healthiest, and fittest life that you can imagine.

VISION BOARD

Similar to the vision board concept attributed to Joyce Schwarz, your wellness vision is a collection of attributes that will complete your wellness journey. How will you look? How will you feel? What will your energy level be? What activities will you enjoy? Collect these attributes to build a mental image of your future self.

As I mentioned earlier, being there for my daughter was my initial *why*. As I created a vision for myself, I realized that I didn't just want to be alive longer; I also wanted to have more experiences with her. Not just watching from the sidelines but actually participating in her life. Let me tell you a little bit about my daughter.

Bekah loves fitness. While most "kids" her age are lying out at the lake or playing video games, she's doing Cross-Fit, killing it on a mud run, or taking a striking class. She's happiest when she's pushing herself. When I committed to staying happy, healthy, and fit, I vowed to be able to participate in those activities with her.

It started with a Warrior Dash, which is a 5K mud run with obstacles. I trained hard, and on race day, I was ready to enjoy it with her. I was living my vision.

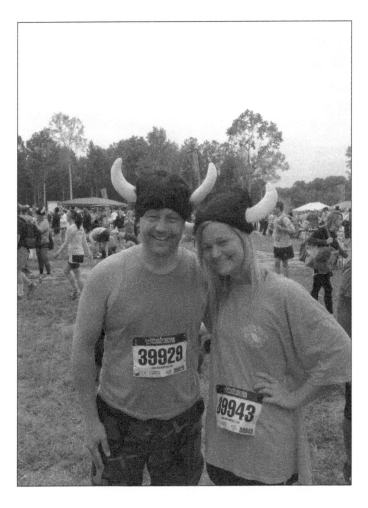

Your vision might start with a very fuzzy image, but I assure you it will get clearer as you go. I started with a Warrior Dash because it was something I was reasonably sure I could do (with some training, of course).

Once I was further along on my wellness journey, and I had run a second Warrior Dash with her, I learned that I had much more physical capacity than I had before. So Bekah and I decided we'd do a Tough Mudder—a *twelve-mile* mud run with obstacles. (I'll share more about that later.)

Earlier, I compared my wellness journey to a drive from Pensacola Beach to Philadelphia. If I didn't have a roadmap or GPS to guide me on that journey, I would likely just start by driving north. That would get me closer to my destination, but my path would be meandering and inefficient.

In order to be efficient on your journey, try to get to as clear a vision as you can and start moving in that direction as early as possible. Like it did for me, your vision will get clearer as you go.

WHY PHILADELPHIA?

In my example of driving to Philly, I picked that city for two reasons: a former colleague I respect is from there, and it's a place I've never been. Your vision should be aspirational and somewhere outside your comfort zone.

COMMITMENT

When you put your *why* and vision together, you have a commitment. I can't emphasize this enough—if you don't commit, you will not succeed at finding true wellness. When you're committed, you do more, you cheat less, and you always know where you're going and why. Through an act of self-love, you have made a vow to yourself.

I encourage my clients to write out their vow and to keep it close at all times. Like a wedding ring, it should be a constant companion on your wellness journey; it will drive every decision. It will help you develop better habits. It will show you the way to a better, healthier lifestyle. It will change you. But it will only do these things if you have a solid *why* and a vision you believe in.

MY VOW

I will put in the time, the effort, and the discipline to obtain good health and fitness so I can enjoy all of the activities that my children, grandchildren, and wife enjoy.

Take your time in making your vow. Make it matter. Then, through self-love, make the commitment to be better for yourself. With that, you now have everything you need to plug the coordinates into your GPS.

I've created a Wellness GPS Workbook with a Vow Worksheet to help you write out your vow. You can download the workbook at wellnessroadmapbook.com/gpsworkbook.

Modern GPS units use an array of satellites to establish where you are in the world. Unfortunately, we don't have software to establish our wellness journey starting point. You'll have to do a bit of work to figure that out for yourself. Let's get going on that.

ESTABLISH YOUR STARTING POINT

As part of onboarding a new client, there are some things I need to know about them. This helps me set a baseline or starting point for their wellness journey. I break these baselines into three categories:

- Medical
- Fitness
- Physique

MEDICAL

Anytime you start a health and fitness lifestyle change, it should include regular visits to your doctor; make her a primary partner in your wellness journey.

A standard checkup will likely include:

- Fasting blood draw
- Weight and/or BMI
- Blood pressure and resting heart rate

- Other standard-of-care tests such as a mammogram, colonoscopy, or prostate exam
- General health questions (my doctor asks about my sleep, stress, energy, and libido)

Most doctors are pigeonholed into a business model that gives them only seven minutes per patient, and most of their patients are there to deal with an illness or injury. Coming to them from a position of wellness might confuse them at first.

Let's go through each of the datasets the doctor takes and consider what it means. This will help you make the most of your seven minutes.

When you make your checkup appointment, the office will often set up a blood draw one morning before your doctor's appointment. I encourage you to get as comprehensive of a blood lab as possible. As you build your wellness roadmap, you'll find tons of value and some great metrics in this data.

Here are some of the health markers your blood draw may have:

- Cholesterol
- Blood sugar
- Stress and cardiovascular risk

- Vitamin and mineral levels
- Hormone levels
- Organ health markers

Every time I go to the doctor, they weigh me. I'm guessing it's the same for you. If you don't fit in the "normal" BMI range, your doctor is likely to tell you to lose some weight. It's the standard of care.

If either your blood pressure or resting heart rate is high, it needs to be addressed. Although the doctor's visit might be triggering the elevation, if you have consistently high blood pressure and resting heart rate, you're putting undue stress on your organs and cardiovascular system. Consider buying a blood pressure cuff and checking it regularly (I have one that connects to my iPhone and records my numbers with an app).

The general standard of care has certain tests coming at recommended ages and at given intervals. I regularly see articles saying that many of these tests aren't necessary, but I'd do what your doctor asks and act accordingly.

Most doctors get into the profession because they want to help people be healthy. Unfortunately, they don't spend much time doing that. As I noted, your wellness visit might surprise them at first, but they'll likely be delighted that you're taking a proactive approach to your health.

Be open and honest with your doctor. Share your vision with them, particularly the parts about health. Ask them what steps you can take to improve your health and wellness. Your doctor won't be your only source of education—you want to seek out knowledge and find out what works for you—but for baseline-setting purposes, you should assume your doctor knows best until you learn otherwise.

FITNESS

In chapter 5, Training, I will be going through various fitness modalities that you can train and improve, but I want to take a moment here to dispel a common myth. This myth is dangerous because it is one of the primary reasons why people quit exercising, especially those of us over forty.

Fitness is not a look. Despite CrossFit's claim to crowning the fittest man and woman on earth, you don't have to look like a CrossFit athlete to be fit. Fitness comes in all shapes and sizes.

Fitness means being able to do the things you want to do.

If you enjoy gardening, you can train to maintain a level of fitness that will allow you to garden. If you enjoy playing tennis, you can train to be a better tennis player. And if you aspire to do something challenging, such as a 5K or a Tough Mudder, you can train to ensure you complete the race with no injuries.

40+ FITNESS SUCCESS STORY

Sue was one of my podcast listeners, and she didn't have astronomical dreams for her fitness. She just wanted to get in and out of her boyfriend's car without any struggle. Sue's boyfriend owns both a 1998 Corvette and a new Navigator. Sue always struggled getting in and out of the Corvette, so she wished he would drive her only in the Navigator.

After participating in the *40+ Fitness Podcast* 28-Day Squat Challenge, she found it so much easier to get in and out of the Corvette. Now she can enjoy driving with the top down without worrying about the in-and-out struggle. She had a vision for what she wanted, which was well within her reach, and she worked to get it.

When you set up your fitness baselines, consider them both in terms of activities you enjoy doing and activities you struggle doing. Knowing where you are now will help you see how your training could improve your fitness and your life.

Struggling to open jars? Building grip strength will help.

Want to keep up with the grandchildren? Endurance training will keep you in the game.

Want to get in and out of a Corvette pain-free? Squats, baby!

PHYSIQUE

I can hear you now: "But, Allan, why would you talk about physique—didn't you say looks don't matter?" Not exactly. What I said was that fitness is not totally based on how you look. Of course all of us want to look good; there is absolutely nothing wrong with wanting that.

Vanity aside, we all want to be more comfortable in our own skin. Here's the good news: you'll likely see improvements in your physique as a result of improving your medical and fitness baselines. But that doesn't mean your vision won't include some work specifically aimed at a better physique.

Wellness is being the happiest, healthiest, and fittest you can be. Looking good goes a long way toward the happiness part. At least it does for me.

THERE ARE TWO WAYS I LIKE TO FIND PHYSIQUE BASELINES FOR MY CLIENTS:

- Before pictures. Just like I did in Puerto Vallarta, take the full front and full side pictures. These pictures don't lie.

- Body measurements. With my clients, I measure the neck, chest, stomach, waist, hips, thighs, and upper arms. In the Wellness GPS Workbook, I've included a male and female chart for you to use. You can get a copy of the workbook at wellnessroadmapbook.com/gpsworkbook.

PUTTING ALL THE BASELINES TOGETHER

When I started training for Tough Mudder, I was already in much better shape than I had been eight years earlier when my journey began in Puerto Vallarta, but I was in no condition to run the twelve-mile race, let alone complete all of the obstacles. These obstacles included climbing, crawling, plunging into ice water, and being shocked by electricity. (Sounds like fun, huh?)

I had to recognize my current level of health and fitness and train hard to get them up to par before the race. I wasn't strong enough, nor did I have the cardiovascular endurance, and I was definitely carrying far too much body fat. That said, I knew the eight months I had was enough time if I stayed true to my commitment.

Then there was Todd, who couldn't exercise at all. What

he could do instead was make some simple nutritional changes that would have major impacts on his health, such as cutting out processed foods and increasing his water intake. Five years into his journey, he's so far away from where he started that he's hardly recognizable as the same man.

TRACKING = SUCCESS

I needed better grip strength to successfully complete the obstacles in Tough Mudder. At first, I tested my grip strength at a personal training studio. I wasn't strong enough to do a single pull-up. But I had a starting point. As you begin your wellness journey, especially if it's your first time ever, no metric is too small or seemingly insignificant as long as it aligns with your vision.

HOW TO CHOOSE YOUR MODE OF TRANSPORTATION

Health and wellness result from your ability to keep moving forward at a pace that best suits you.

My brother, John, is a brewmaster in Asheville, North Carolina. You think when I visit him I'm not going to drink his beer? Don't be silly! I have the mindset that allows for detours, so I take that into account as I structure my lifestyle. That's my baggage.

An honest assessment of the baggage and the passengers

you're bringing on this journey will help you figure out what type of vehicle you need.

Do you want to get to your final destination quickly? Maybe you have a high school reunion coming up or you've signed up for a 5K in two months' time. Then you might hop in a sports car and head out. The sports car goes fast and handles well when the road is open and clear. For the eight months I was training for Tough Mudder, I singularly focused and drove hard and fast. Fortunately, things fell into place and I was able to successfully complete the race. But I know that pace is just not sustainable for long periods.

I love going to Southern Miss football games in Hattiesburg, Mississippi, which is only three hours from where I live. I know the route so well I don't even think about it when I'm driving. I could use a fast car with the single focus of getting there at a quick but reasonable speed (yes, I have gotten a speeding ticket driving to a game; what can I say?).

But what if I want to set up a tailgate? Then I have a lot of baggage to carry with me, such as the tent, grill, food, water, beer, and so on. That baggage changes the vehicle I'll need to use. With all of the tailgating supplies, I'll have to sacrifice my speed for something that can haul all of it, such as my pickup truck.

That's the same way I think about wellness. If I have a body composition goal that I want to reach, then I might hop in that Ferrari and let 'er rip, despite the risks. However, when I prioritize happiness as an element of wellness, I'm willing to slow down my journey, as long as I'm still moving forward. (For the record, I don't own a Ferrari.)

"I GOTTA GO PEE"

As you work to understand the right pace for your wellness journey, you might find you have some passengers. A spouse, kids, friends—all of whom can change how you go about your journey. Notice how I didn't say they can change your vision. You are the only one who can control your vision, regardless of who accompanies you.

Never forget, **you are the driver on your wellness journey.**

Start by being honest with yourself. Then be honest with the passengers. Tell your friends and family what you need from them. You might say, "I'm about to change the way I eat and exercise. How can we structure our meals and free time to do this in a way that makes all of us happy?" Then listen in earnest.

Honesty—with yourself and the people closest to you—is

the key to grounding yourself. You need to know what you want for yourself so you can tell them how you need your food prepared. If you don't eat starches, and you're surrounded by people who do, you'll need a plan for how to avoid them.

Even if you're not all working to get to the same destination, it's important that the people closest to you—your spouse and kids—understand why you're building this roadmap and, at the very least, don't hinder you from reaching your vision. I would encourage you to share your vow with them (very likely, they're a big part of your *why*).

I'd like to share a quote by Parker J. Palmer, and I really want you to meditate on it: "Anytime we can listen to our true self and give it the care it requires, we do it not only for ourselves but for the many others whose lives we touch."

You *need* to make this journey. It is going to make you a better spouse, a better parent, and a better friend.

TAP INTO YOUR EMOTION

Perhaps like Todd, your journey will force you to face some harsh truths you've been avoiding for a long time. That's the value of grounding yourself in why you're going on this journey in the first place.

You're a human being. There's no surer way to yo-yo back and forth between health and unhealth than by not having a solid, emotionally driven commitment that drives you down the road to wellness. This lifestyle change will come from your core.

Dare to dream. Then make the investment of time, effort, and money to make it happen. It won't be easy, but it certainly will be worth it. Wellness on your terms is one of the greatest joys in life. The life I've lived since I committed to wellness is so much better than before. That's why I have dedicated myself to helping other people find their vision.

Even if you don't have a brush with death like Todd did, you still have a desire for something better for your life—that's why you're reading this book. And behind that desire is an emotion. Tap into that emotion in order to make your wellness a reality.

After working through this chapter, you've now given the GPS your starting coordinates and your destination. We all start from where we are and need to get somewhere different. Your wellness journey is unique to you. You'll only reach your destination by grounding yourself firmly in reality, without shying away from the best you're capable of and the challenges you'll likely face to get there.

In the next chapter, we'll get familiar with the route we're going to take on our wellness journey. We'll learn to look at the journey as a series of mile markers and how these mile markers keep us focused on moving forward and showing us the progress we're making as we get there.

CHAPTER 2

PERSONALIZATION

Bekah and I went back to Puerto Vallarta in 2009. I was fitter now, and I was beyond excited for us to play beach volleyball together. There'd be no subbing out this time.

Normally, there would be anywhere from four to six people on each side, but for one reason or another, it was just Bekah and me. Luis (the guy who'd taken my picture) and another vendor showed up and wanted to play us. I hadn't played two-man beach volleyball in nearly fifteen years, but we really wanted to play, so I agreed.

If you know beach volleyball, you know it's not the easiest sport in the world. It's two constant battles: one between you and the opponent, and another between you and the sand. I sweat my ass off playing that game, but my training kept me playing nevertheless.

Bekah and I gave them quite the game. I don't recall the final score, but it was down to the wire. More importantly, I was spending fun, fitness-oriented time with my daughter. The commitment I'd made to be a better father was coming to life. I felt that my heart might burst—not from exhaustion, like the last time I tried to play, but from sheer joy.

That day was all the proof I needed that having a solid commitment based in self-love is the key. I was living my vision of wellness.

That day was a turning point for me. It showed me that I'd already traveled through a major section of my wellness roadmap. The accomplishment and joy of that game left me with a great sense of clarity. If I kept myself on the track toward my vision, nothing could stop me. And I was so ready to tackle the next section of my roadmap.

CREATURES OF HABIT

We are creatures of habit. Unless there's a traffic accident or road closure due to construction, we'll get up in the morning and drive to work the same way we always do. Everyone in your office probably does the same thing, too.

However, here's the difference: even if we have the same job, our drive to work will be different because although we're going to the same place, we live in different houses. Therefore, we start in different places.

That example illustrates one of the main problems in using a one-size-fits-all diet or workout program, and it's why I don't advocate them: you need personalization for your plan based on your unique combination of starting and end points.

Even though I describe portions of the wellness journey as segments or mile markers, please don't think there are short-term fixes. Building true wellness requires us to change our lifestyle. Breaking the journey into mile markers makes the task easier. How do you eat an elephant? One bite at a time.

THE VISION FROM THE MOUNTAINS

My friend John and I moved to the same county in Mississippi during the eighth grade. In a small high school where everybody knew everybody, John and I were the guys who talked funny. We played football together. We both had blond hair. Now we both shave our heads. And strangely enough, we both married women named Tammy.

Thirty years after high school, both John and I ballooned out in size. John managed to remain jolly, whereas I went the bastard route. I'm not entirely sure how it came to pass, but John and I formed a team to run what was going to be my second Warrior Dash with my daughter. We went all out on this one (at least from a wardrobe perspective).

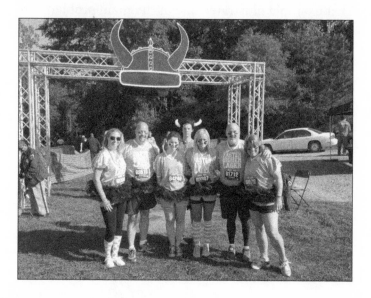

SAY NO TO THE TUTU

Special note: Don't wear a tutu on a mud run; it catches on the barbed wire, and if you don't keep your arms up, they'll chafe.

Up until this point, most of my wellness roadmap had been focused on building the fitness necessary to do the things Bekah and I enjoyed doing, such as volleyball and Warrior Dashes. So I was plenty fit to complete the race. But even as we did this second one, I weighed about 240 pounds and had 37 percent body fat.

Once I started training for Tough Mudder, I knew I had to do more than just build strength and endurance. I needed to lose body fat. As the result of changes I'd made in my eating (including doing Paleo and keto) and the work I was putting in at the gym, I was closer to 205 pounds and 19 percent body fat on race day.

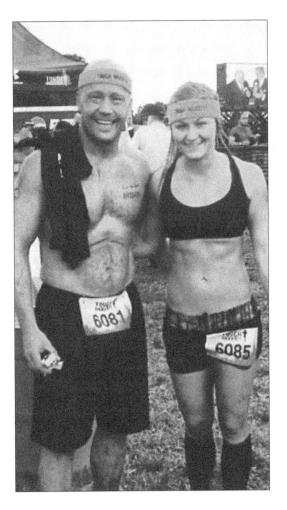

John saw my picture on Facebook and messaged me to ask what I had done. He asked me for help. I told him I didn't mind taking him on as an online client—I'd be happy to help an old friend—but in order to make his lifestyle change last, I also wanted to train his wife, Tammy. I knew I wouldn't be able to meet him in the gym every day, so in order to make his changes stick, he had to have another source of accountability. Tammy needed to be on the journey with him.

John had a knee injury from high school that we had to work around. But he was able to pick up without nearly as much trouble as Tammy, who had back issues. They were starting at different places, but they both had the same vision: they wanted to move to the mountains of Tennessee and enjoy hikes in the wilderness.

Although they wanted to get to the same place, we had to personalize their roadmaps to take them on different routes.

It was understandably distressing for Tammy whenever her back went out and she was stuck in the bed for days at a time. My role as her trainer in those moments was to reinforce to her that she could get on the road to Tennessee, even if everything she'd ever read told her she couldn't burn enough calories to lose weight without exercising.

I worked with John and Tammy for ten weeks. We had weekly conversations (some of which we recorded for the podcast), and over the course of those ten weeks, John lost thirty-nine pounds and Tammy lost twenty-eight pounds. Of course, weight loss wasn't the only indicator of success they were going for, but they knew they were closer to their goals.

They're not yet ready for retirement, but because they each followed a personalized plan, John and Tammy now live in Nashville, Tennessee, exactly where they wanted to be, enjoying the beauty of nature they dreamed of.

MILE MARKERS

Everything is driven by your original vision. For John and Tammy, it was their dream to retire in Tennessee. For me, I want to continue being active with my daughter. I want to be there as she grows up, ready to play beach volleyball whenever we can.

I also want to maintain my independence. I want to be able to wipe my own butt when I turn 105. I know that sounds pretty peculiar, but you'd be blown away by how many people lose their independence after seventy because they didn't maintain their health in their forties and fifties.

As I mentioned earlier, we break down our roadmap into sections or mile markers. Another name for these are goals. More specifically, I like to use SMART (Specific, Measurable, Attainable, Relevant, and Timebound) goals because, by their very nature, they will align to your vision. If your GPS tells you to drive 1.3 miles and turn left, that's your goal for the next couple of minutes. Each SMART goal you set will bring you closer to your vision.

HOW TO CREATE SMART GOALS

SPECIFIC

Your SMART goal needs to be very distinct so you know the next mile marker you're driving toward. By making your goal specific, you can determine indisputably whether or not you've reached it. I find that when people make their goal ambiguous and hard to define, they do it out of fear—if you aren't specific, you won't know when you've failed. It's a defense mechanism.

For example, let's say my SMART goal is to look like Vin Diesel. I'm already a bald muscular guy, so I have a head start, but what's wrong with this goal? Why isn't it SMART? Well, first of all, I don't know how healthy Vin Diesel is. I can look at a picture of him and figure he's a pretty strong guy, but I don't know his underlying health profile. What's his blood pressure? What's his body fat percentage? Can he run five miles? Because I don't know the answers to these questions, there's nothing specific for me to strive for.

Looking like Vin Diesel didn't align with John's vision either. Nothing about having huge arms and a huge chest would improve his chance of hiking the mountains of Tennessee with his wife.

Moreover, the end result is subjective—to some people, I may already resemble Vin Diesel. How will I determine which day I look enough like him to say I've reached this goal? Your SMART goal has to be specific.

Because John was prediabetic, one of his SMART goals was to get off his medications. By being so specific, he was very close to hitting that mile marker after just ten weeks of working together.

MEASURABLE

If you can measure some aspect of your goal with objective numbers and accomplishments, you're more likely to achieve it. Fitting into a dress two sizes smaller, getting your waist down below forty inches, and completing a 5K are all measurable goals. You can track your progress over time.

A lot of people use weight as their goal measurement—"I

want to lose twenty-five pounds"—because it's easy to track. I've already discussed why weight is not a great health or fitness marker. Just because something is easy to measure doesn't make it a good SMART goal. Focus your goals on the markers that can be measured and directly affect your happiness, health, or fitness. Rather than trying to lose weight, you're better off focusing on reducing your stomach circumference, as that does have a direct correlation to cardiovascular health risk.

If John's goal is to get off his meds, his doctor needs to see an A1C level (a measure of blood sugar) of less than 6.0. By tracking his A1C levels, he has a measurement that is directly related to his goal.

ATTAINABLE

Your SMART goal is doomed from the beginning if it's not realistically possible. Growing up, my dream was to play in the NFL. I trained hard and had a great high school football career. But my size and, in all honesty, my skills didn't match up to what I needed to take that next step. Once I knew this goal wasn't attainable, I shifted my efforts toward more appropriate pursuits.

I've always had good endurance. Knowing this strength, I was confident that if I was willing to train hard enough, I could do a Tough Mudder with my daughter. That's not to say you should pick goals that are only in areas of your strengths—not at all. If you do choose a SMART goal in an area where you're weak, make sure it's not so high-reaching that it's unattainable.

I didn't set my first goal to run a Tough Mudder. Instead, I worked to do a couple of Warrior Dashes first. They were attainable and gave me the confidence to stretch myself.

RELEVANT

Your SMART goal has to be tied to your vision. I've gotten off my roadmap plenty of times. I once trained for a Spartan race. I was working hard on strength and endurance, but as my strength started to climb, I became distracted with the desire to get my deadlift up to five hundred pounds. For some reason, that seemed really important to me at the time, but how did a five-hundred-pound deadlift improve my chance of completing a Spartan race? How did it get me toward my vision of being there for my daughter as a healthy, happy, fit father throughout her life?

As a result, I went on a detour on my road to wellness. I didn't get to five hundred pounds on deadlift. I got really close, but I didn't have the final push to make it happen, because it wasn't relevant.

TIMEBOUND

A goal without a deadline is a wish.

If you don't have a deadline, you won't be fired up to get anything done. When I signed up for Tough Mudder in March 2013, I knew I had only until November to get ready for that race. I bought race entries for Bekah and myself because I was committed to that deadline.

Your deadline should be less than a year, preferably a quarter or a month. Longer-term goals often die on the vine. If you are really stretching yourself and need more than three months, you may want to break the goal into smaller subgoals. Goal setting is a skill, and as you get more practice and a better understanding of your body and mind, you'll get more comfortable setting appropriate deadlines.

Some of the best deadlines are those that fit naturally into our lives. Maybe your daughter is getting married in four months and you want to drop two dress sizes. Or you want to be ready to spend time with your grandchildren when they come to visit you over summer break. June will be here before you know it, so you'd better get started making this goal a reality.

You'll find the SMART Goals worksheet in the Wellness GPS Workbook at wellnessroadmapbook.com/gpsworkbook.

Whether it was playing volleyball, running obstacle course races, or doing CrossFit, I made sure all of my SMART goals led to my spending more active time with my daughter. The SMART goals might have changed depending on her interests, but the vow and the vision would remain the same.

Breaking your larger vision into smaller SMART goals makes it easier to wrap your head around a potentially long journey down the road.

SH*T HAPPENS

Forrest Gump is one of my favorite movies. In one scene, when Forrest is running, he steps in some dog poo. The guy running beside him makes a big scene about it. Forrest simply replied, "It happens." We all step in dog poo sometimes, and Forrest Gump's response is a perfect example for you on your wellness journey.

You can avoid most of the dog poo you step in by having no more than three SMART goals at a time, and maybe just one at the beginning. If you try to start eating a ketogenic diet, train for a 5K, and start a squat challenge all at the same time, you're setting yourself up for failure. Pick only one and make it happen.

Make your SMART goals matter. Let's say you learn that

intravenous vitamin C is a wonderful health intervention. That's great, but if you're still eating processed garbage food, a boost in vitamin C won't do you much good. Instead of setting a goal to get a shot every week, set an aligned SMART goal to cut out the processed foods. You'll likely get all of the vitamin C you need from the whole foods you're eating.

Use SMART goals to incrementally build a platform for even greater successes. After I had completed two Warrior Dashes with Bekah, I had an excellent platform from which to aim for a Tough Mudder. Having that base level of accomplishment gave me the confidence that I could continue progressing.

CHECK THE EGO

Don't let your ego goad you into setting SMART goals that are not smart. In 1995, while going through a divorce, I started training for a marathon, and I set my sights on running a hundred-mile race. I was twenty-nine years old and in great shape. I completed five marathons that year.

Then I signed up for my first ultramarathon. It was nearly twice as long as a regular marathon (fifty miles) and on trails instead of roads. I did finish the fifty miles, but after achieving that, I realized there was no reason to put my body through another race that length, let alone something twice as long. It was more likely to break me than to help me. Unlike my deadlift debacle, that was an instance where I recognized that goal was leading me away from wellness.

Occasionally, you're going to mess up and step in some poo. Just shake it off and press on to another mile marker. A slip is only a failure if you quit.

PUSH YOURSELF—TO A LIMIT

You have to know who you are in order to stretch yourself the appropriate amount beyond your comfort zone. Too far and you'll discourage or break yourself; not far enough and you won't progress at the rate you could.

Finding your limit is a function of honing the self-awareness to see yourself objectively. Even with self-awareness, we all screw up sometimes. At least that's what happened to me as I watched infomercials one Sunday morning.

CHAPTER 3

SELF-AWARENESS

It was a Sunday morning in early 2010. Work had me traveling about 90 percent of the time, so I was taking full advantage of a rare weekend at home, resting everything but my thumb. I was sprawled out on the couch flipping between *Face the Nation* and weekend infomercials.

An advertisement popped up for the Insanity workout with Shaun T. I leaned forward on the couch—the man looked amazing. All the people behind him were exercising as he coached, and they looked great, too. They were sweating, they were happy, and they were fit.

I was five years removed from my *decision* in Puerto Vallarta, and I was at an ebb in my wellness journey, rather than a flow. I was marginally fitter than I'd been back then, but I could feel my momentum fading. Weeks on the road for work meant I wasn't exercising regularly.

And because the Insanity workouts didn't require equipment, it seemed perfect for me.

I called the toll-free number and bought the DVD set.

When the DVDs arrived, I opened the box like a child opening a Christmas present. I spread the DVDs and booklets out on my kitchen counter to take it all in. They had meal plans, protein shakes for sale, and about a dozen DVDs with the workouts. I popped in the first DVD and pushed my couch out of the way to make room for my Insanity.

The first step was taking a guided test, meant to gauge my fitness level. I was so hyped that I hit that test as hard as I could. I quickly jumped in different patterns, did squats, and lunged all over my living room. Physically, I was capable of the movements, but I could tell within the first minute that this was going to be very difficult.

After the test, I was lying on the floor huffing and puffing, just like the Insanity crew on the DVD. I was tired but extremely proud of how hard I had worked. I showered and went about my business.

The next morning, I opened my eyes and I felt like I'd been strapped to my bed and beaten with a baseball bat—I couldn't move. I take that back: I could raise my arms a little, but it hurt so bad I didn't want to. I tried to get up for work, but it was not happening—I couldn't get out of the bed. I thought back to the team behind Shaun T. I doubt they woke up like me the next morning.

I couldn't imagine sitting at my desk all day in so much pain that I wouldn't be able to concentrate on work. Everyone would wonder what the hell was wrong with me as I walked around the office like a mummy.

What I had was something called delayed onset muscle soreness (DOMS), which is not life-threatening but hurts like hell. I do not handle failure well, and this felt like a huge fitness failure. At my age, my mind hadn't caught up to my body.

DELAYED ONSET MUSCLE SORENESS

Delayed onset muscle soreness (DOMS) is a common experience during resistance training, especially when you start new exercises. DOMS is a very acute muscle pain, but it is not an injury. If you get a case of DOMS, be sure to drink plenty of water and try to keep moving the affected muscles throughout the day. In time, the pain will subside.

Just remember, DOMS is neither a good thing nor a bad thing. It is just an indicator that you pushed yourself. But you should not make DOMS a goal. You are still making progress, even if you don't get DOMS.

That moment in bed, totally incapacitated, is a big reason why I focus my podcast and personal training on people over forty: by the time we reach that age, our capacities are lower than in our twenties. We now have to deal with our past injuries or the effects of sitting at a desk for twenty-plus years. It's hard for our youth-seeking minds to catch up to our aging bodies.

My mind had pushed my body past what it was capable of doing in that moment. I overdid it so badly that I had to call in sick for work. My inclination to go from the couch to standing behind Shaun T on the Insanity DVD absolutely sabotaged my decisions to improve my fitness.

I never did a single workout from Insanity—I'm guessing those videos are still somewhere in my house, but I seldom think about them. Even though I'd be able to do them now, I lack the desire, all because I pushed too hard when I didn't have the self-awareness to realize I didn't need to.

DON'T PASS THE RED LINE

If I didn't put my ego in the back seat, I was never going to get to my wellness destination. I would only continue dealing with DOMS, or worse, injuring myself. I could blame Shaun T, but I know who did this to me: I did.

It's easy to laugh about it now, but that was a turning point for me that easily could have gone the other way. If I had never learned to stay within my capacity and only pushed hard, I would have burned myself out and potentially given up the entire journey.

Think of an old car: if you just step on the accelerator without easing up, you'll redline the vehicle and you might blow the engine. Likewise, if you have worn-out brakes (your knees), you won't want to follow the car in front of you too closely. If you understand the capacity of your vehicle, you'll be more likely to get from point A to point B in a responsible and efficient way.

We're not twenty years old anymore, and most of us aren't driving new sports cars. Take it easy on the accelerator. There are few things worse than redlining over the age of forty and injuring yourself. It's harder now than ever to recover. This can really set you back, especially if training is a big part of reaching your vision.

After my incident with the Insanity workout, it took me years to learn how to stay within my capacity and manage my ego. I also learned the value of consistency and progression. It was a painful lesson I learned from my overzealous participation in the Insanity workout—or, rather, the Insanity fitness test, because I never made it to the actual workouts.

CHILDLIKE MOBILITY

If you're a prudent driver, you take your car in for a diagnostic check before you hit the road for a long trip. Otherwise, you risk breaking down and waiting on the side of the road for a tow truck. You need to do the same for yourself before you start your wellness journey.

Understand what your injuries and choices in the past have done to your body and how they affect you today. Because of years sitting at a desk, I know I have certain muscle imbalance. Take an inventory of what your lifestyle has done to your body over the years. Before you get started on this journey, you might have to get corrective surgery or start physical therapy.

This is an important part of your wellness journey, and you shouldn't take it lightly.

Most of us have nagging injuries. I'm not just referring to the popping, stiffness, and pain we feel in the morning. What I'm referring to is even more serious than that. One in five people over the age of seventy has a tear in their shoulder, and one in three people over ninety years old has a tear.[3] We develop these injuries because most people over forty have what corrective exercise defines

---

3   L. Nové-Josserand, G. Walch, P. Adeleine, and P. Courpron, "Effect of Age on the Natural History of the Shoulder: A Clinical and Radiological Study in the Elderly," *Revue de Chirurgie Orthopedique et Reparatrice de l'Appareil Moteur* 91, no. 6 (2005): 508–514, https://www.ncbi. nlm.nih.gov/pubmed/16327686.

as movement compensations. You walk, run, or otherwise move in an unnatural pattern to account for pain or muscle imbalances.

When we were kids we'd sit cross-legged for story time. When was the last time you tried to sit cross-legged on the floor?

We've been sitting in chairs for decades, so we don't have the mobility to comfortably sit on the ground anymore. Once they got us out of kindergarten, they stuck us in chairs and we've been sitting in them ever since: from our desk at work to the wheelchair in the nursing home.

Have you ever watched a child squat? They look so natural and comfortable squatting down to pick up a ball and hopping up to run away with it. As adults, even in our twenties, we have already made lifestyle choices—such as sitting for long periods or wearing high heels—that inhibit our natural movement patterns.

We'll talk more about mobility in chapter 5, Training, but I want to stress here that it is critical that you identify your physical limitations and work on fixing them *before* you set out on your fitness training. Just as driving a car that isn't properly aligned will wear out the tires quickly, you need to get your body aligned before you start pushing yourself. Our bodies are machines, after all: they can and will break down.

MENTAL SELF-ASSESSMENT

Taking stock of your physical starting point is important, but what about your mental strengths and weaknesses? You've committed to a wellness journey, but what if your kids still want to eat Oreos and ice cream? What if your spouse wants to eat out three nights a week? Will you have the mental capacity to maintain your path and account for potential detours?

Identify your potential sticking points and how to compensate for them. Where have you slipped up in the past? What caused you to quit on an exercise plan or cheat on a diet? Do you know how to say no when someone brings doughnuts to the office staff meeting?

Be realistic—lying to yourself by thinking you can avoid all temptations is not a good approach to wellness. Remember that wellness is being the happiest, healthiest, and fittest you can be. Being miserable and depriving yourself is not going to cut it. Detours happen. By knowing when and why you're taking a detour, you'll have more control over it.

Having mental self-awareness is much more difficult than having physical self-awareness. You know where your aches and pains are physically; you feel them when you walk down the stairs or squat down to pick up a child. But we are so good at lying to ourselves about our mental tenacity. You won't succeed if you're not honest with yourself.

BUILD A TOOL KIT OF HABITS

Build out a tool kit of habits and strategies that help you stay the course. Learning from my own mistakes, I found that if I want to work out at lunchtime, I need to pack my gym bag the night before and leave it by the door. If I don't, I'm liable to forget my workout clothes or shoes. Packing the bag and leaving it where I'll trip over it on my way out the door ensures I have no excuses.

It's the *mental* blind spots that will force you off the road on this journey. Once you get those dialed in better, you'll see improvements in your fitness and understand yourself even better. That's the only way to build the wellness lifestyle you want.

SABOTEURS

As you work through the self-awareness stage of your Wellness GPS, you'll recognize saboteurs. Saboteurs come in all forms—ranging from evil to well-meaning.

EVIL SABOTEUR

This is the person who will bring a doughnut by your cube and say, "Hey, I grabbed you a doughnut so you don't miss out."

You respond, "You know I'm eating low-carb to be healthier. We had this conversation last week."

Then she flippantly says, "It's just one doughnut."

That's the saboteur who doesn't want you to succeed. They're trying to undermine your efforts intentionally to see you fail. They're the ones who will tell you your nutrition plan will make you die of heart disease or that you're doing something terrible to kill your metabolism. "You'll go into starvation mode," they'll say.

They'll focus on the negative aspects of your life improvements. No matter how amazing your coworkers, friends, and family are, there will be a few people who just want you to fail.

They don't want you to change because your success highlights their failure. Keeping the status quo helps them stay in their comfort zone. Misery loves company. You have to either separate yourself from these people or flat-out ignore them. Stay the course. Don't let them bring you down.

THE WELL-MEANING SABOTEUR

These are the people who truly love you and really want to be positive influences on your life, but they simply believe what you're doing is terrible. They don't tell you you're hurting yourself because they want you to fail; they worry about you hurting yourself, even if they're wrong.

These interactions are difficult because these people genuinely care about you, and you should keep them in your life, but what they're doing is going to inadvertently sabotage your efforts if you allow it to.

This saboteur also comes in the form of a friend inviting you out for a few drinks to "catch up."

They mean well, whether it seems like it or not. That's just their lifestyle. It used to be your lifestyle, too, but you have to ask yourself if you can maintain those same lifestyle choices and still fit them into what you want for your vision.

As well-meaning as those people might be, or as close friends as they are, you may just have to say goodbye to them (if only for a short while). At the very least, tell them that you're not going to interact with them in the same environment anymore. If they want to hang out, they'll have to do it on your terms.

If you know you'll have difficulty avoiding drinking martinis at the bar, you can say, "The bar doesn't interest me, but how about we meet at the park after work tomorrow and go for a walk?"

It's not easy, but if they can't meet you where you are in your wellness journey, then you may have to distance yourself from saboteurs, even the well-meaning ones.

MINDSET

As you adapt to your new lifestyle, you'll start forming different and better habits. Suddenly, you'll be eating healthier, moving more, sleeping longer, and having a better outlook on life. You'll feel more energetic, and that will drive you to even more change.

I'd encourage you to focus on changing one or two habits at a time, especially when you first get started. It's easy to get overwhelmed when you're making too many changes at once.

If you start off by saying you want to cut out processed foods, stop drinking alcohol, do a couch-to-5K program, start sleeping eight hours a night, meditate every morning, and journal every day, that's a recipe for distraction. It's like having your GPS in your car telling you to turn left, your spouse telling you to turn right, and your back-seat passenger telling you to stay straight. Trying to go in so many directions at once will cause you to ignore your Wellness GPS, and you'll fall back on decisions and willpower—and we all know where that leads us.

STACKING HABITS

In the Surefire Results for Weight Loss program, I work with clients over the course of twenty-eight days to implement three simple habits: eat less sugar, drink more water, and take up a daily walking routine. All of these habits stack onto each other very nicely, and I'm there to guide them along the way so my clients get results.

(Yes, I do call it a weight loss program, but that's only because nobody looks for a fat loss program. As the marketing adage goes, "Sell them what they want, and give them what they need." The lost weight is just a side effect of the fat they lose.)

Make sure your mindset is focused on just a few habits at a time to reach your next mile marker. Each mile marker you reach will teach you about yourself and give you much more resilience, making it easier to see your way to the next mile marker. It's like getting the right prescription for your driving eyeglasses: now you can read the signs and know you're on the right track.

MINDFULNESS

How do you handle stressful events in your life? What would happen if, after building habits and reaching your

SMART goals over time, you injured yourself? Or suppose you got into a car accident? How would that impact your mentality? Would you feel defeated and then regress?

While I can only guess at your response to these hypothetical setbacks, they're worth thinking about. Only so much is under your control. You might have a setback—you're human. This is where mindfulness becomes the best navigator you could ask for.

Mindfulness allows us to be present, but it also helps us manage our response to outside influences. Staying mindful helps you see the speed bump and slow the car down.

If you can predict how particular events will trigger stress and anger for you, you can better prepare for them when they happen. I've had high-stress jobs, and I learned that rather than turning to booze, I can take it out on the weights in the gym. That time could have easily been spent in the bar after work, but through mindfulness I recognized the pattern and made the change in my life to use it for my wellness.

BACK TO INSANITY

I had good intentions when I tried Insanity, but as you've heard, the road to hell is paved with good intentions. I went into that workout (well, fitness test) with plenty of passion but no strategies to back it up. "But look at all those people in the infomercial! They're in great shape. I'm in good hands." The testimonials, the packaged set, the diet plans—I knew it had to work. However, I didn't know that my body *wasn't* capable of doing it, and that seriously impeded my progress—I went over a speed bump way too fast and it put my car in the shop. Then I let that moment of discouragement stop me, and my wellness declined as a result.

Shaun T couldn't see me pushing too hard; he couldn't tell me to back down. My GPS was set beyond my capabilities, and I suffered for it. Good intentions and bad application sent me down the wrong path because I lacked self-awareness.

Now that you've learned how to practice self-awareness, you've successfully set your GPS. You know where you're going (you have a vision) and the reason for the trip (you know your *why*). You've laid out your personalized course for your wellness roadmap, and you can see your first mile marker (your SMART goal). You also know your car is fit for the journey (meaning you've assessed your mental and physical capabilities and limitations). And your driving glasses (mindfulness) are smudge-free. You're ready to go!

It bears repeating: you are the driver on your wellness

journey. So turn that ignition. Let's take it to the STREETS and see where this journey takes us.

PART 2

———

STREETS

Once you have your GPS coordinates set, you still have a lot to figure out on the road. Where are the best places to stop for gas? What is the speed limit on your current stretch of highway? When should you set the cruise control?

In this section, I'll help you with the Strategies, Training, Rest, Energy, Education, Time, and Stress Management to get you to your wellness destination.

You need a user manual for your life—one that won't be like anyone else's, because we weren't made on a factory assembly line. As you learn and build out your user manual in part 2, you'll be better equipped to operate your vehicle and continue down the road to wellness.

I would love to tell you that the road is all clear—that there are no detours, no construction zones, and no storms to slow you down. But that's not the case. Some jackknifed trailer truck could back up traffic for hours. Rain will make the roads slick. And road construction could force you off the highway and through a dangerous part of town. A million little problems will pop up to detour and slow you on this journey you're taking toward your vision.

My goal is to help you handle the obstacles with ease.

CHAPTER 4

STRATEGIES

From the outside, your and another person's wellness journeys might look identical—you might even cruise down the same road for a while. But inevitably, if your visions are different, your paths will diverge. That's what happened with two of my clients, Trent and Rich, who often find themselves in very similar circumstances but have extremely different wellness goals.

Both Trent and Rich have jobs and family lives that require regular travel, and they face distinct challenges on the road, both with exercise and nutrition. So what can they do on the road? Do I just tell them to suck it up for a few days and accept that it's a lost week?

No. We set up a strategy *beforehand* to find solutions to common issues that have a tendency of derailing them.

When Trent first came to me as a client, he was already going to the gym regularly, but he wasn't seeing the results he wanted. He enjoyed hour-long runs because they helped him deal with stress. Unfortunately, many of the foods he liked weren't the right foods to meet his body composition goals. He struggled to add foods that would help him. Being on the road made his food choices that much more difficult.

Rich, on the other hand, was far from a gym rat. He preferred working out at home or being in the fresh air, pounding the pavement, or on a trail through the woods. Rich absolutely loved all food. He was an adventurous eater, always willing to try new things. Because of his eating habits, although he was fairly active, he still couldn't lose body fat.

When their respective coworkers and clients went out for dinners on the road, Rich wanted to eat everything on the menu. Trent, being a picky eater, struggled to find food that fit his tastes, so he either under-ate or made poor choices on the road.

With Trent, I encouraged him to bring food on the road and keep it in his room, just in case the conference meals didn't fit his nutritional needs. With Rich, I coached him to drink a glass of water before going to dinner and another glass while he waited for his meal. That way, his water intake would keep him from overeating.

In either case, I told them to do research on the areas they traveled to in order to find gyms, running trails, grocery stores, and restaurants with healthy options.

Trent and Rich were different clients facing different wellness obstacles under similar circumstances. Both wanted to change their body compositions by losing body fat and gaining muscle. Although on the surface you might expect their journeys to follow the same road, they needed vastly different strategies for dealing with their unique obstacles. The key to building wellness strategies is doing what works best for you.

OOPS!

Thinking back to the self-awareness you gained in chapter 3, what are some upcoming speed bumps that could decommission you in the near future? You have headlights on your car to see ahead, but you still have to drive defensively to ensure you don't hit anything. Your goal is to look at the week ahead and see if there are any obstacles that you will need to avoid or traverse.

SPEED BUMPS

What is the number one excuse most people use when they aren't meeting their health and fitness goals?

I'm too busy.

You wouldn't be too busy to pick up your spouse from the airport, would you? You love them, after all. You'd make time for him no matter what. So why do you think it's OK to use busyness as an excuse not to show yourself love?

To reach your wellness goal, you have to prepare. For example, you might believe you don't have time to cook healthy meals each night, so you need effective strategies to traverse that speed bump, such as batch cooking on the weekends. (I'll get more into food in chapter 7, Energy.)

Likewise, if you know you're about to do eighteen-hour workdays, you may have to change your fitness schedule. What can you do to get your fitness training in? Do a high-intensity interval training session, which takes less time, instead of a longer cardio session. Also, you could switch your strength workout to a bodyweight workout so you don't have to bother driving to the gym.

Maybe your best friend's birthday party is on Friday and you know everyone will be eating cake and drinking wine. What is your strategy for that day? How will you manage your food intake over the course of the week to either account for the cake and wine or avoid them?

Perhaps you know ahead of time that the party will be at

a restaurant. You can look up the menu online and see what healthy options they have available. If they don't have any, you may choose to eat at home beforehand and drink a large glass of water before you arrive.

Most speed bumps have a warning so you can slow down. Take time to consider what speed bumps are coming your way this next week. Then develop and repeat strategies to account for each one. There is no excuse to bottom out your car when the signs are there. You just have to look out for them and plan accordingly.

WHERE SELF-AWARENESS MEETS STRATEGY

Can you be in the company of people eating cake and not partake? Or do you know you'll want to eat some, too? Either feeling is valid, but you have to recognize which is more likely for you so you can prepare accordingly. Even though I've weaned myself off sugar and I can easily decline cake, if I know cake will be around, I'll bring some seeds or nuts so I won't be the only one not eating. This strategy makes the interaction less awkward for everyone, and it helps me stay on my wellness path.

ALIGNMENT

Although your headlights improve your line of sight down the road, you will never see all of the obstacles in front of you. But if your strategies are aligned to your vision, you can compensate for the most common obstacles, and you'll be more likely to traverse them. No matter how well you know yourself, you'll still run into moments with surprising triggers that make you fall into bad habits and bad new behaviors.

Imagine your gym closes for a month due to renovations. Will you still find a way to work out at home, or will you give in and take the month off?

I've seen people leave their road to wellness because of potholes like that. They do a U-turn and go right back to where they started. But you made a commitment, remember? You have to work through the roadblock with a shift in strategy.

Where I used to work in South Arkansas, there was an amazing doughnut shop called Spudnuts, where they made their doughnuts out of potato flour. When someone brought Spudnuts to the office, it was like sharks being chummed. I'll admit, they were delicious, so Spudnuts were a huge pothole for me.

When you hit that first pothole, you recognize the road is more treacherous than you'd expected. You have to slow down and keep your eyes peeled, just in case any other potholes pop up on the road. I mitigated the Spudnuts risk by keeping bags of nuts and seeds in my desk and avoiding the break room when Spudnuts were around.

While getting around roadblocks and avoiding potholes might seem like a demonstration of willpower, it's actually not. It still goes back to your commitment based on self-love. You know your vision and your *why*. You made your vow to your health the same way you'd make a vow to your spouse.

If an attractive person started flirting with you, would you automatically be disloyal to your spouse? Of course not! You made a vow.

Your health is far too precious to cheat on.

ADJUSTMENTS

In 1991, I attended a corporate manager training session in Jackson, Mississippi. When we returned from lunch one day, every table had three buckets and a jar. The jar was empty, but the buckets were each full: one had big rocks, one had little rocks, and the final bucket had sand. The instructor tasked every table with a seemingly impossible task: fit all of the rocks and sand into the jar. We struggled for about twenty minutes before he finally stopped us. Looking around the room, I could see that nobody had succeeded.

"This is impossible," one of the trainees spoke out.

The instructor told us that it was indeed possible to fit

the contents of the buckets into the jars. We just had to be intentional about how we did it. He demonstrated the proper strategy by carefully placing the big rocks into his jar first. Then he slowly poured the little rocks in, and shook the jar to let them settle in the cracks between the bigger rocks. Then he poured in the sand and shook even more vigorously. The sand settled into every nook and cranny left in the jar.

Like magic, he'd fit every big rock, little rock, and grain of sand into the jar, simply by starting with the big rocks first.

The lesson was clear: you have a limited amount of time and energy, so you have to focus on the big things first. Likewise, you should first focus on making the big-rock adjustments that will give you an opportunity to let the smaller adjustments fill in the cracks.

DETERMINING YOUR BIG ROCKS

How do you determine which adjustments make up your big rocks?

It all comes back to your vision. My vision required me to get stronger, build endurance, and lose body fat. To get stronger, I had to lift heavy things. That was my first big rock in the jar. In the beginning of my journey, there was no reason for me to worry about supplements such as creatine, pre-workout energy drinks, or protein shakes—those were little rocks and sand. I just needed to learn good form for each exercise and then start adding weight as I gained strength.

For the endurance, I just laced up my running shoes and hit the road. When the weather was bad, I wore out the elliptical at the gym. I wasn't looking for sugary gels, complex training regimens, or altitude masks, because those were all small rocks that would just distract me. My biggest endurance rock was to simply start moving progressively farther and faster.

In order to cut down my body fat, my biggest rock was my food choices. I started eating Paleo because it made sense to me, and it seemed sustainable. I used Mark Sisson's Primal Blueprint as a guide. During those first few weeks, I would dream about bread, but rather than looking for a recipe for Paleo bread, I kept my focus on my big rock: eating a diet with mostly meat and veggies.

As you work your way through the remainder of the STREETS part of this book, try to find your big rocks. Making those adjustments will get you moving quickly and safely toward your vision. Your body will tell you when it's time to start adding the little rocks and then the sand, but for now, your strategy should always have you focused on the next biggest rock.

ACCOUNTABILITY

Be strong, be fearless, be beautiful. And believe that anything is possible when you have the right people there to support you.

—MISTY COPELAND

As I mentioned in the introduction, we wear a wedding ring for multiple reasons. Yes, we wear it as a symbol of our bond to our spouse, but we also wear it to announce to the world that we're taken. It's an outward sign that we're not available, we're in a committed relationship, and we will never break our vow.

We should be just as outwardly loyal to our health journey. You should have no hesitation telling someone you're working to correct your health, so you won't be able to participate in their unhealthy activities. The biggest determinant of whether your social circle supports your lifestyle changes will be your communication of your *why*.

In a study published in the *Journal of Personality and Social Psychology*,[4] the researchers observed people's behavior in line at the copier. They went through a series of asking people in line if they could go ahead of them. They asked in three different ways:

---

4   Susan Weinschenik, "The Power of the Word 'Because' to Get People to Do Stuff," *Psychology Today*, https://www.psychologytoday.com/us/blog/brain-wise/201310/the-power-the-word-because-get-people-do-stuff.

- "Excuse me. I have five pages. May I use the Xerox machine?"
- "Excuse me. I have five pages. May I use the Xerox machine, because I have to make copies?"
- "Excuse me. I have five pages. May I use the Xerox machine, because I'm in a rush?"

What do you think was the percentage of people who complied with each request to break in line?

- Sixty percent of people let them break in line when they were asked the first prompt.
- Ninety-three percent of people let them break in line with the second prompt.
- Ninety-four percent of people let them break in line with the third prompt.

In other words, the use of the word *because* resulted in more people willing to help. If you want someone to help you, you need to give him or her a reason. Your *why* isn't only important for you—your friends and family want to know it, too. Be sure to share it!

If you say you want to lose weight so you can run a 5K with your daughter, you've made your goal more personal, and your social circle will be much more likely to support you and hold you accountable.

Fixing your health and holding yourself publicly accountable might feel like it opens you up to embarrassment and ridicule. I understand that it's not easy to tell people you're making a change in your life. And while I can appreciate your concerns, it is time for you to get past that. Take those rose-colored glasses off and see things for how they are.

You have only one body, and it isn't getting any younger.

ACCOUNTABILITY TEAM

If your social circle loves you, they'll be on your team. Even if they understand what you're doing, don't expect all of them to change their own habits.

Despite my best efforts over the years to get her to quit, my half-sister still smokes. She also eats crap food. It's a shame, because her father (my stepfather) died of a heart attack at forty-seven. Even though I know she loves me, I can't expect her support on my wellness journey.

I want you to realize something important: even if the people closest to you are not supportive or don't understand this journey, there *are* people out there who are interested in finding training partners, walking buddies, or accountability partners to share in the journey.

Find them through online communities such as the 40+

Fitness Podcast and MyFitnessPal. Also, many online communities are based on different ways of eating, such as ketogenicforums.com or veganforum.org. And, of course, there are Facebook groups with like-minded people discussing any wellness topic you want to learn about.

Most gyms hold group workouts, or you could try a boot camp class. I play beach volleyball on a recreational league team, and I'm sure you could find a local sport and level that suits you. I've even seen people advertise for walking buddies on a neighborhood classified website.

Opportunities to find accountability are all around you.

HOLDING YOU ACCOUNTABLE WITHOUT KNOWING IT?

I had an interesting conversation about accountability with a client. He goes to the gym at the same time each day and sees the same people there. While he hasn't formed a friendship with any of them, he still thinks of them being at the gym on the days he misses, which encourages him to show up on the days when he doesn't want to.

When I was a teenager, my friends and I would pile into cars and cruise Delaware Avenue from one end of town to the other. Why did we do that? We did it because convoys meant we had a community with us. It made for a more fun and inclusive experience. You're less likely to pull off the road and go somewhere else if several other vehicles are expecting you to keep up.

That's the same reason we have training buddies. Because it's hard to go on this journey alone, no matter how fun and exciting it can be. Having accountability partners—whether in the form of teammates, loved ones, or even trainers—can make you more likely to reach your destination.

HIRING A COACH OR TRAINER

The mediocre teacher tells. The good teacher explains. The superior teacher demonstrates. The great teacher inspires.

—WILLIAM ARTHUR WARD

When you first learned how to drive, did you get behind the wheel all by yourself and hit the road immediately? (Well, I grew up in the country, so that's what some of my friends did, but that's beside the point.) For most people, the answer is no. You had someone sitting in the passenger seat, telling you what to do as you learned. They not only kept you from driving too fast, but they also helped you learn how to operate the car and understand the rules of the road.

That's the same support a fitness coach or trainer can give you: they help you learn faster than you would on your own.

A good coach is helpful at any juncture on your wellness journey, but they are *most* beneficial at two points: the beginning of the journey and when you reach the cusp of excellence.

The coach you have at the beginning will tell you what to do, how often to do it, and when to rest. The same way a driving coach helps you operate the car safely, a good coach will ensure you use good form and don't wreck yourself.

You probably already know how to drive, so you don't *need* to hire a driving coach. But you might change your mind if you were to buy a new BMW with a stick shift—nobody wants to be grinding gears on an expensive car.

As you improve your health, your body will become more like the BMW you don't want to damage. Your coach or trainer is tasked with helping you keep your car in excellent condition—that's an important job. Don't just accept the trainer the gym wants to assign to you; pick the one who is best for you. Here are the traits I look for when I hire a coach.

SPECIALIZATION

A coach who tries to coach everybody can't coach anybody.

Michael Phelps is an Olympic swimmer. He doesn't need

a powerlifting coach or a running coach. He needs a swimming coach, and he might need a specialized swimming coach at that. He's so good that he needs to refine techniques to a microlevel that most of us will never reach in any given modality.

Although you won't need someone as specialized as Michael Phelps would, you still need to choose your coach based on their specialty. Do they focus on strength or physique? What about your age group? We'll talk about the various training modalities in the next chapter, and once you know which modalities matter most to you, you'll have a better idea of what coaching specialization you need.

CURIOUS

A good coach will have a lot of questions for you. They will want to know:

- Who you are
- Your goals
- Your past training experiences
- Your physical and medical limitations
- How often you can train

When they take those factors into account, they will give you advice based on your specific needs. If they pull out a fixed program from a filing cabinet without asking about you and your goals, they are not likely to be a good coach for you. You want a coach who really listens to you and treats your best interests as a priority.

SET YOUR COACH UP FOR SUCCESS

Most people who hire a trainer at the gym choose weight loss as their primary goal. It's no wonder trainers get numb to the *real* needs of new clients, then find it easier to hand them fixed workouts. Tell them your SMART goals so they can be the coach you need them to be.

If you walk in the front door of the gym to meet with a personal trainer and they *don't* ask you about your vision (in so many words) or why you're doing what you do, then move on and find someone else.

A bad trainer, without curiosity, assumes that every client is driving the same car down the same road toward the same destination. That's just not how it works.

PERSONALITY

I was a military kid, and I was in the military myself. Having someone yell at me actually makes me move faster. Now, they don't have to be mean about it, but being coached by someone who's aggressive actually works well for me. You might like the same thing.

My driver's ed teacher, Coach Bennett, was also my offensive line coach in high school. What was cool about him was how he could go from whistle-blowing, yelling football coach to calm, nurturing driver's ed teacher. He was a great coach for me on the field and behind the wheel.

Do you want the forceful coach to push you harder? Or is it the more empathetic coach who will best suit you? Most coaches have one style or the other. Great coaches like Coach Bennett know when to be forceful and when to be empathetic.

I didn't get to choose Coach Bennett, but you do get to decide whom you work with as a fitness coach. It can be difficult to discern the training personality of your potential coach, so don't be shy about telling them what you're after and asking if they can be that person.

Most of your time during a training session will be spent talking about the work at hand, your weight for the next set, and comments on your form, but there will be times between sets when other aspects of your lives will come up in conversation.

Before you hire a trainer, ask yourself: Is this someone I'd like to spend multiple hours talking to each and every week? The teaching time could be great, but if the rest of your time together is uncomfortable silence, how will that go? If you don't like your coach's personality, the resulting friction can become an easy excuse to skip training sessions or, worse, quit altogether.

EDUCATOR

When your father, mother, sister, or whoever taught you how to drive, did they just get behind the wheel and tell you what to do while you sat in the passenger seat? They might have at first, but if they were any good, they let you drive yourself and taught you the basics as you went along. Then you got your driver's license and continued on without your coach.

The reason you were able to move on was because they taught you lessons and pushed you to be good enough to go on your own. They let you get behind the wheel yourself. Your coach should approach your health and fitness the same way.

Their mindset should be, "How can I coach myself out of a job?" At some point, they should want you to know what you're doing, why you're doing it, and how you're doing it to the point that you don't need them anymore. The last thing you want is a codependent relationship with your trainer.

WHEN TO FIRE A COACH

Client turnover is part of a personal trainer's life.

For bad trainers, it happens when they are not giving their client what they need and that client finally does the cost-benefit analysis and moves on. Money and effort aside, your time is too valuable to waste on a bad trainer. You deserve better.

Even if you have a good trainer, you might reach a fitness level that requires you to get a higher-level coach.

Michael Phelps doesn't have the same coach as he did when he first started swimming. He had to find progressively better coaches and, in many cases, *teams* of coaches to address every facet of his work. You may love your coach, but you may eventually realize it's time to move on.

There are four main reasons to fire a coach.

They're Actually a Bad Trainer

We all get pressured to make purchasing decisions we don't actually want. When shopping for a trainer, you may have made the decision after a thirty-minute consult without realizing you'd made a mistake. If you finish your first session with your new trainer and you realize you aren't a good fit together, you have two options:

1. Ask the gym if you can switch to a different trainer (which can create an awkward scene).
2. Train through your prepurchased sessions and change trainers at that point.

Something Changes in Their Life

Your trainer is human. As a result, they will experience negative life events, and through no fault of their own, they might lose focus. Maybe they're dealing with family problems, they have too many clients, or they're just burned out (which happens with a lot of trainers).

Because you'll likely have a personal relationship with

your trainer, you should feel comfortable asking them what's going on if they don't seem present. Their issue might be temporary. My trainer, Dave, wasn't himself at one of our sessions. It turns out he'd broken up with his long-term girlfriend. He was back to being Coach Dave the next week. If your relationship isn't something you see turning around, you can tell them you're stepping back, charting your own course, and going your own way.

Something Changes in Your Vision

In this case, you might have your own life event, or you simply want to take a different path. For example, what would you do if a DEXA scan showed you were at risk for osteoporosis? Would you stay on the same course, or would you make changes in your wellness roadmap? That might be a time to move on from your running coach because you want to focus on lifting with heavier weights in order to strengthen your bones, rather than focusing on a 10K personal record.

They Have Nothing More to Teach You

The final major circumstance in which to let go of a coach is when they've taught you everything you need to know and you can either go it alone or hire a better coach. This is the ideal situation and what I work toward with all of my clients. I hope they'll stay for my charming personality, but if I've gotten them as far as I can, I understand when it's time for them to spread their wings and fly.

BECOME UNRECOGNIZABLE

We travel through our wellness roadmaps by having strategies. These strategies are aligned to our vision, which ensures we continue moving in the right direction. There may be setbacks where you have to make adjustments, but we have to have faith in ourselves that we will reach our vision. An accountability team can be a big help in keeping that faith.

Rich is on a wellness journey that is dotted with speed bumps and potholes, along with the occasional planned detour. To many people, he might be moving slowly, but he knows exactly where he's going and how to get there.

Trent's road isn't any easier than Rich's, but he highlights another side of strategy: it's important to have one, but you must *execute* it to make it worth anything. When Trent reached an intermediate level with his health, I asked him if he would be game for a program that required more gym time. He was up for it, and now he's in the gym more and showing great results.

After months of setting and executing on strategies aligned to his vision, Trent went to the gym for one of his training sessions. The woman at the front desk did a double take when he handed over his ID.

"Sir," she said, "I'm afraid we can't allow you to use another member's ID card."

That's how different he looked: the man standing before her was so much fitter and trimmer than the man in the ID image that he had become unrecognizable.

You don't know everything that will happen on the road to wellness, but you can train yourself to be better equipped for the journey. It starts with a strategy that you execute. As speed bumps and potential detours pop up, you need to become a defensive driver, regroup, and restrategize. And onward you go!

CHAPTER 5

TRAINING

I need to put one thing out there right now: you must *train* your body to be well and stay well—it won't happen otherwise.

There, I said it.

Each of us is on an aging curve. While some of the effects of aging are outside our control (like genetics and serious injuries), the rate of decline caused by aging is most highly influenced by the lifestyle choices we make. In other words, you choose how fast your body ages.

If you don't train, you're choosing to age faster. I don't think that is the wellness vision you have for yourself. So how do we change how we age?

HITTING THE SLOPES AT NINETY

I interviewed one gentleman for the *40+ Fitness Podcast* named Fred Bartlett, an Army Ranger who, at eighty-six years old, is still a hard-driving attorney.

Despite his gung-ho mentality, when Fred reached age fifty, his girlfriend (now wife) woke him up to the fact that he was not on the right health and fitness path. At that moment, he created a new vision for himself: Fred was an avid skier, and he still wanted to be on the slopes at age ninety. He made a commitment and vowed to himself that he would finally take care of his wellness.

Fred now watches what he eats, and he also lifts weights and stays active. He knows that when he doesn't train, he's sending a message to his body that it can decline at whatever rate it wants. Now, even though he's older than he was when he made his commitment, he is the driver on his wellness journey, and he refuses to let his body decline against his will.

Each year after he made his commitment, Fred went on ski trips with his buddies. They had a blast carving down the mountains together.

While they all enjoyed those trips and wanted to come back, nobody but Fred truly committed to a vision of going skiing every year for the rest of their lives. At every skiing trip thereafter, the group dwindled. Fred watched as his friends got too old to participate.

Fred, on the other hand, stayed on the Strong Path, as he calls it—he refused to become too feeble to ski. He might get old, he told himself, but he would never become feeble, and he would not stop skiing.

Now, at eighty-six years old, Fred carves down the slopes past people half his age, still enjoying his life while his friends are all at home or passed away.

Although there is a road that most people go down, you can choose a different road. You can use the tools I'm about to share with you to live your vision, and like Fred, you can add both years to your life and life to your years.

Contrast Fred with my grandfather, who had given up on his passion, golf, before he turned eighty. He is now well into his nineties. He's alive, but he's lost his independence, which truly breaks my heart. It was also a huge wake-up call for me. If I want my independence at his age (i.e., being able to wipe my own butt at 105), I need to train for it.

Until scientists crack the code to the fountain of youth, we'll have to settle for the next best thing: training. To reach your vision, you'll have to train. You have to press the gas pedal if you expect to move forward.

DISEASE AND MOVEMENT

Disease is the opposite of wellness. Most of the diseases people are getting today—such as heart disease, diabetes, and some cancers—are caused by our lifestyle choices. These diseases were very rare a hundred years ago. Some people blame processed foods, soft drinks, and fast food, but I think an overlooked contributor is lack of movement.

Just as cars went from hand crank to key ignition to push-button start, our lives have gotten more and more convenient. (I'm sure we'll eventually be saying something like, "Siri, start the car.") As our lives have gotten physically easier, we've become more sedentary.

Until recent history, getting food alone was serious work, whether it was hunting and gathering or working a family farm. The US Department of Health and Human Services recommends that adults get at least 150 minutes of moderate exercise per week. That may seem adequate, but I doubt our ancestors could get a week's worth of food in two and a half hours—we've set the bar really low.

MOVEMENT AND YOUR LYMPH SYSTEM

Beyond the physical signs of health that come from a good training regimen, we need movement to rid our bodies of toxins. The lymph system is the highway for shuttling toxins from the cells out of the body. Whereas the lungs rely on the diaphragm muscle, and the heart is a muscle, the lymph nodes don't have muscles specifically for pumping toxins. They rely on skeletal muscles (those that make us move) to force the toxins through the system. When we're immobile, toxins can build up in our lymph system and cause issues.

We are all starting at different points. I had a guest on the *40+ Fitness Podcast* named Lorraine. When she first started, she couldn't walk up her driveway without stopping to rest multiple times. Two years later, she was in the gym regularly and moving along in her wellness journey.

The lesson is that it's never too late to start. With proper training, anyone can improve their fitness. Now, that's work with a payoff.

In the following sections, I'll describe the various fitness modalities that you can focus on in training. I'll help you align the modalities that best fit your vision, and I'll give you some general advice to get you started.

BODY COMPOSITION

Most people start their wellness journey with the idea that weight loss equals health. As I've stated before, that's just not true. I want you to change that mindset by focusing on your body composition, meaning you build muscle, give yourself stronger bones, and *potentially* lose some body fat. (If you haven't settled your mind on the big picture of body composition, please go back to chapter 1, Grounding.)

THE THREE ELEMENTS OF GOOD BODY COMPOSITION

A good body composition requires three changes:

1. More muscle (more weight)
2. Denser bones (more weight)
3. Lower body fat (possibly less weight)

When two out of the three side effects of being healthy and looking better actually require you to gain weight, do you see why weight loss is not the right metric to prioritize?

Let's take a moment to discuss the three elements of body composition and why they matter to you.

MUSCLE

One of the sad, hard facts about aging is that in lieu of training, we will lose about 1 percent of our muscle mass per year after the age of thirty-five. It's called sarcopenia. That loss accelerates after the age of sixty-five.[5] I'm guessing you can do the math in your head. A large portion of the muscle you have will be gone by the time you're seventy-five.

I'm sure you've seen this happen to people: they dwindle into smaller and feebler versions of their younger selves, and quite frankly, it's sad. And the worst news is that muscle helps protect bones from breaking when we fall. Muscle acts as a cushion. With lower muscle mass comes a higher likelihood of broken bones, especially after falls. Victims of sarcopenia don't just look feeble, they are feeble.

It's very sad indeed because sarcopenia can be prevented. All it takes is some resistance training (which I'll explain more about in a moment).

---

5   Mary E. Sehl and F. Eugene Yates, "Kinetics of Human Aging: Rates of Senescence between Ages 30 and 70 Years in Healthy People," *The Journals of Gerontology: Series A* 56, no. 1 (2001): B198–B208, https://academic.oup.com/biomedgerontology/article/56/5/B198/554581.

BONES

Let me introduce you to sarcopenia's twin sister, osteopenia. Most of the ladies reading this book will already know this one. Osteopenia is the consistent loss of bone density, and it also starts to take effect around age thirty-five. Similar to sarcopenia, osteopenia works at a rate of 1 percent per year. Together, they are a deadly one-two punch that destroys body composition and causes us to become old and frail.

While getting proper calcium and magnesium in your diet is important for maintaining healthy bones, the best way to increase bone density is—drumroll please—resistance training. Just as your muscles gain mass from training, your bones gain density through the same process, which helps you simultaneously stave off both sarcopenia and osteopenia.

BODY FAT

A healthy body has *some* body fat. In fact, many of the bodybuilders and elite marathon runners with extremely low body fat have significant health issues. But all that said, with the current obesity rates, most of us could stand to shed some fat.

We carry body fat for two reasons: to provide fuel when food is scarce and to keep us warm in cold weather.

Because we live in a world with an abundant food supply and we spend most of our time in climate-controlled environments, having excess body fat isn't necessary. Instead, we should strive for a healthy balance.

In general, a woman over forty should have between 19 and 35 percent body fat, and a man over forty should have between 9 and 25 percent body fat. Those may seem like wide ranges, depending on where your body stores fat, but you can narrow them down. If you carry your fat on your stomach, you're at a higher risk of cardiovascular disease, so you might be better served by pushing your body to the lower end of your suggested range. If your body fat is on your hips, you can live toward the higher end of the range and enjoy those healthy curves.

How do you train to lose body fat? The answer is you don't. You lose body fat based on what and how much you *eat*. You can lose body fat while training for other modalities, but you just can't depend on training alone to cut fat. (We'll talk more about nutrition in chapter 7, Energy.)

ALL THE PARTS

Our total body weight is mostly composed of muscle, bone, body fat, and water. So when you step on a scale, it will tell you the total weight of all elements combined, but not the relative percentage of each element.

There are various ways to assess body composition besides weight. Let's take a moment to discuss each one.

BODY MASS INDEX

Everybody loves shortcuts. Beyond weight, the next most popular estimate of good body composition is the body mass index (BMI). Your BMI is a calculation that uses your weight and your height, and is only marginally better than weight as a tool for understanding body composition. (I dislike this formula so much that I'm not going to bother sharing it with you here.)

According to my BMI, I was classified as overweight, at 28.6, when I did Tough Mudder with my daughter. My body fat was less than 19 percent, but my BMI indicated that I should lose more weight (muscle, bone, fat—where the weight comes from makes no difference when calculating BMI). For most people, BMI can be a quick and easy tool to track trends, so long as you know you're not sacrificing muscle or bone to get to a result.

BODY MEASUREMENTS

I was driving across the flat portion of Colorado, and it was mind-numbingly absent of landmarks. I drove (faster than I should have) and it didn't feel like I was getting anywhere. Knowing how that feels, I make sure my clients have a quick and easy way to monitor progress. Do that with body measurements. With a simple three-dollar cloth tape measure, we can get a good idea of whether we're making progress.

With my clients, we measure:

- Neck
- Chest at the thickest part
- Stomach at the belly button
- Waist at the thinnest part
- Hips at the thickest part
- Each thigh at the thickest part
- Each of the upper arms at the thickest part

The GPS Worksheet at wellnessroadmapbook.com/gpsworkbook has a male and female diagram for you to record your body measurements. You can print out several of these, and by measuring yourself over time, you can track trends in your body composition change.

ELECTRICAL IMPEDANCE AND CALIPERS

If I worked with my clients in person, I could use tools like electrical impedance or fat measurement calipers to get a slightly better fix on fat percentage. These tools, while marginally better than body measurements, are not foolproof—tracking trends is the key.

DEXA SCAN

In my opinion, if you really want to know where you stand from a body composition perspective, you can't beat the DEXA Scan. It is similar to an MRI (although you're not encased in a claustrophobic tube). It takes a series of scans of your body over the course of ten minutes. It measures your bone density, muscle mass, water, and the fat in every part of your body. While it can be expensive, the data will tell you exactly where you stand in terms of body composition. I get one about every two years.

Your body composition is going to be a result of two factors: your nutrition (which we'll discuss further in chapter 7, Energy) and your lean body mass (meaning muscle and bone).

STRENGTH

Have you ever struggled to open a jar? You're then resigned to ask for help or do without. You've just experienced a loss of independence due to strength loss. Just as we lose muscle to sarcopenia, strength declines at about the same rate.

What may start with jar lids that are "too tight" will soon be grandchildren who are too big to be held, and then not having the leg strength to stand from a seated position. It is a gradual decline, which is how it sneaks up on you.

How much joy do you feel picking up a child—whether your own, a grandchild, or someone else's? It's an amazing moment of connection to bend over and pick them up. What if you're so weak you can't pick them up? Isn't it worth dedicating some time and effort to maintain the strength to do that?

I mentioned getting up from a seated position. What if that seated position involves a toilet? Sure, you could have rails installed, but in time, even that won't be enough. Isn't it worth dedicating some time and effort to keep up your strength?

Maybe this conversation is a bit uncomfortable. Good. I'm fairly certain your vision doesn't include losing things that bring you joy. I am also sure you want to maintain independence for as long as possible.

Furthermore, studies have shown a huge correlation between grip strength and longevity. I think grip strength is an excellent and underutilized indicator of overall health. We all remember our grandfathers, or maybe our fathers, who had that wiry strength, where they didn't look like they had much meat on them, but man, when they shook your hand, you could feel their innate strength like a vise wrapping around your palm. That's because they worked hard and did things with their hands all day. We called that "farm-boy strong."

You're not going to get hands like that sitting at a computer clicking a mouse all day or swiping at your phone screen.

Beyond the changes in the work we do, people have invented some great gadgets to help us with our strength dilemma: rails for the toilet and bathtub, chairs that lift up to help us stand, and grippers to help us open jars. In theory, they're great—they extend our timeline of independence—but as we become dependent on them, they also make us decline faster.

Choose resistance over the easy route.

Have I convinced you that you need to train for strength? Good, let's get started.

RESISTANCE TRAINING

Just as you will increase muscle mass and bone density with resistance training, you will also increase strength. It is a wonderful gift to have a body that, when stressed by resistance, can adapt and grow more muscle mass, build bone density, and get stronger. Don't shun that gift. Start a resistance program ASAP.

You'll often hear resistance training referred to as weight lifting. Now, before you panic, thinking about hernia-inducing, backbreaking, knee-destroying exercises with rusty iron bars and tons of weight plates, stop. Take a deep breath. You already have all the weight you need to get stronger: *your body.*

Moving your body weight is enough to get stronger for most people, especially if you haven't done much resistance training lately. How many body weight squats can you do? What about push-ups? Pull-ups? Those exercises use your body, the simplest and most cost-efficient weight system available to you. So don't assume you have to buy a weight vest or dumbbells all of a sudden; leave that for later.

Investments in equipment or a gym membership may come later as you progress, but they aren't absolutely necessary to get results early on.

WHAT ABOUT THE GYM?

You don't have to go to a gym or build your own weight room to do strength training. I'll share some of the pros and cons of bodyweight exercises versus home equipment and a commercial gym:

TYPE	PROS	CONS
Bodyweight	Free	Can be boring after a while
	Can do anywhere	
		Progressions can be difficult
	More forgiving on form	
Home Equipment	Convenience	Can get expensive
	Buy as you progress	Takes up space
	Some variety	Lifting weights alone can be dangerous
Gym	Low monthly rates	Not as convenient
	They look after the equipment	Busy gym times/ Equipment taken
	Lots of variety	Other people's sweat and germs
	We work harder around others	Can feel intimidating
	Other gym services, including Personal training	

THE ELEMENTS OF A GOOD STRENGTH TRAINING PROGRAM

- Good form
- Adequate resistance
- Adequate rest and nutrition
- Appropriate progression

GOOD FORM

At first, the term might seem a bit nebulous—what on earth does *good form* mean? In a basic sense, it means moving your body the way it was meant to move. You've probably heard the same sage advice before you picked up something heavy: "Don't lift with your back—use your legs." That advice is prompting you to use good form.

For reasons I'll go into in the mobility section, when you move the way your body is designed to move, you protect yourself from injury. The converse is also true: bad form will hurt you.

You can think of good form in the same way you think of seat belts: it should be second nature. It's the first law of resistance training. Learn good form. Practice good form. It is a nonnegotiable of training.

Teaching you good form is one of the biggest benefits of working with a personal trainer. Yes, you can watch YouTube videos to see how the exercises are done, but a trainer will point out subtle issues that could lead to injury later.

MACHINES VERSUS FREE WEIGHTS

Is one better than the other? Under the right circumstances, both free weights and machine exercises have their value. Machine exercises are very easy to learn: there is usually a diagram on the machine showing which muscles are being worked. Machine exercises move your body along a linear and fixed pathway, which can restrict range of motion. You're also less likely to drop the weight on yourself because the weights are never over your body while you're lifting. It is for these reasons that machines are a bit safer than free weights.

However, when your granddaughter runs up to you and asks to be picked up, you don't lift her in a fixed movement—there's no specific path. Free weights will make you stronger, not only in the muscles that cause the movement but also in the stabilizing muscles. Free weights will give you better functional strength.

If you're a beginner and don't have a trainer to teach you good form or you're rehabbing an injury, then machines can be a good tool to get you stronger. But I strongly encourage you to use free weights in your resistance training. Start with very light weights, learn the form, and progress from there.

ADEQUATE RESISTANCE

For your body to change, it must be *gently nudged* to do so. The resistance should just stress your system enough, and that stimulus will get a reaction: growth and strength improvement.

You may recall my Insanity workout story from chapter 3, Self-Awareness. I pushed myself too hard and paid the price. Conversely, curling three-pound dumbbells won't stress your muscles enough to prompt any progress.

Many of my clients use resistance bands, for which I'll often prescribe three sets of ten repetitions. They should struggle with that routine, particularly on the last set. If they can easily do the three sets of ten with a given band, then we didn't have enough resistance.

Push yourself hard, but don't let your ego break you.

ADEQUATE REST AND NUTRITION

When we do resistance training, we are causing our muscles to break down. That breakdown allows the muscle to rebuild, and when it does, it will come back stronger. That is, if we give it the time and nutrition to do so.

A muscle can usually rebuild itself in thirty-six to forty-eight hours (there are exceptions, such as the core muscles, but this applies to all of the muscles you'll train for strength). If you're working a body part more often than that, it won't fully recover and you won't be getting the full benefit from the work you do. Instead, take time to rest and use your time to do other things, like walking, mobility work, or tai chi (we'll go deeper into rest in chapter 6, Rest).

Your muscles are made of protein, so if you're not getting enough protein in your diet, the muscle won't have what it needs to rebuild. But don't go hog wild on protein either—it's hard on your kidneys. Most nutritional experts recommend 1 to 1.5 grams of protein per kilogram of lean body mass. If you're training hard, I'd target the top of that range. (We'll talk more about nutrition, including protein, in chapter 7, Energy.)

OVERTRAINING

As you progress in your training, you will usually add volume to your workouts by either training for longer sessions or by doing more sessions per week. For example, if you're a runner, your mileage will increase over time, and you'll reach a point where your training will—despite the feel-good endorphins—become a major stressor. If you keep pushing yourself beyond that stress, you can reach a state of overtraining.

For the beginner, it is highly unlikely that you'll do enough volume in your workouts to worry about overtraining, but you should still pay attention to your progress and understand that there is a middle ground at which you're still improving your fitness and not overstressing your body.

APPROPRIATE PROGRESSION

After some time at a given resistance, you'll reach a strength level where that resistance no longer challenges you. Sadly, I've seen many people in the gym who keep using the same weights, workout after workout, month after month. It's sad because they're not getting any stronger or adding any muscle mass.

To get stronger, you have to continually increase the resistance (meaning you lift heavier weights). This is called progression, which you should do in only small increments. Keep good form and you'll see your strength improve.

KISS: KEEP IT SUPER-SIMPLE

Strength training programs range from very simple to ultracomplex. Start on the simple end of the spectrum. I typically recommend a resistance training routine of five exercises (body weight squats, side lunges, push-ups, band rows, and overhead band presses) for which the only equipment you'll need is a set of resistance bands. I would do five sets of five repetitions with sixty seconds of rest between each set.

MOBILITY

Mobility is the capacity to move a joint through its full range of motion.

We lose mobility due to two phenomena: injuries and muscle imbalances.

When we injure ligaments and tendons in a joint, scar tissue forms. Even though the injury heals, we may still lose some mobility due to that scar tissue. When I was thirty-one, I turned my ankle landing from a jump during a volleyball game. I was sure it was broken—even the doctor thought so—but the X-ray showed no break. It was a very, very bad sprain. With medical care and physical therapy, I was back on my feet and playing volleyball again a few weeks later, but the scar tissue that resulted from that injury reduced the range of motion in my right ankle.

The other precursor to lost mobility, muscle imbalance, has two common causes: either we move a joint in a repetitive manner or we don't move it enough. In our sedentary lifestyle, we find ourselves sitting most of the day. As a result of all this sitting, our hip flexors shorten and tighten, and we don't engage our buttocks as much as we should. The result is a muscle imbalance that makes squatting with good form difficult. When you're getting up from a chair with no arms do you tend to lean forward first? That's a result of muscle imbalance.

Aside from sitting, another common practice reduces our mobility: wearing high-heeled shoes. Ladies, I know why you're doing it, but they shorten your calf muscles, which causes an imbalance in your lower body.

Without mobility, the things we enjoy—such as taking walks, going to the zoo, or playing tennis—transform from enjoyable activities to painful experiences we'd rather avoid.

Children squat and run naturally, almost as a compulsion, because they have full functional fitness mobility. However, we've let time and lifestyle choices take that mobility from us. Without good mobility, we are susceptible to injury because we aren't able to use good form, even in our normal daily activities, such as picking up a bag of groceries or stepping into a bathtub.

Before I do any programming for my one-on-one clients, I take them through a movement pattern test. It's pretty simple, really: I videotape them doing a squat with their arms over their head. If their knees collapse in or their upper body leans forward in the squat, I know there's an imbalance somewhere. Ninety-nine percent of the time, this imbalance is a result of tightness in their calves. This small lack of mobility in the ankle works through their body like a chain breaking the natural movement pattern, which, if not addressed, will lead to injury during training.

There are a few things we can do on our own to address tight, shortened muscles such as our calves and hip flexors. These protocols include:

- Self-myofascial release (SMR)
- Static stretching
- Dynamic stretching

SELF-MYOFASCIAL RELEASE

SMR, otherwise known as rolling, uses devices such as foam rollers, lacrosse balls, and specialized rolling pins to release muscle tension. Our muscles are equipped with a safety mechanism that keeps them from being pulled apart (I know that sounds gory, but stick with me). When a muscle is put under too much pressure (which manifests as tightness), this mechanism will make the muscle relax.

I have very tight calves. When I press one of my calves against a foam roller, it hurts. If I press down a little harder and hold it for thirty to sixty seconds, the muscle relaxes. With a few minutes of finding pain points and pressing them, I can get my calves to relax and my range of motion in my ankles improves dramatically.

Note that while SMR is also called rolling, the point is not to just roll the muscle. You're finding points of tightness (pain points) and pressing to make the muscle release. If you just roll over the muscle, you're missing the value of the exercise.

STATIC STRETCHING

Whereas SMR helps to release your muscles, stretching helps to lengthen them. In static stretching, you're placing resistance against a single tight muscle, but rather than trying to fight the resistance, you let it lengthen the muscle. You should hold static stretches anywhere from thirty seconds to a minute.

Because I've spent so much time sitting (especially while I'm writing this book), I like to stretch my hip flexors. One of my go-to stretches is a deep squat, where I squat down until my butt is nearly touching the ground and I hold that for about a minute. I may get some strange looks, like when I did it in an airport terminal after a fifteen-hour flight, but it sure does make me feel (and move) better.

NOTE ABOUT STATIC STRETCHING

Studies have shown that statically stretched muscles have impaired strength immediately after stretching. If you're going to do strength training, you may want to avoid statically stretching the muscles requiring strength.

DYNAMIC STRETCHING

Unlike static stretching, dynamic stretching does not appear to impair strength. In dynamic stretching, you move through the full range of motion, becoming more forceful as you go. If you've ever watched professional athletes warm up before a game, you've seen them bound around to stretch their bodies, rather than focusing on static, isolated movements.

I will use dynamic stretching when I'm about to play a sport, such as volleyball or tennis. Again, dealing with my sitting affliction, I want to open up my hips and stretch my hamstrings. I'll usually do some Samson lunges followed by some jogging movements like high knees and butt kickers. Not only does this warm up the muscles I'm about to use, but it also improves my range of motion and helps me avoid injury.

OTHER MOBILITY PROTOCOLS

There are times when SMR and stretching aren't enough, particularly when you're dealing with an injury. When that's the case, you may want to hire a physical therapist to help you. They may choose one or more of the following protocols:

- Flossing: With flossing, you use a strong rubber band to move the bone around a joint capsule. This is often used when there is scar tissue from a previous injury impairing joint movement.

- Graston Technique: With this technique, also known as gua sha, a therapist uses an instrument to scrape at the scar tissue around a joint. This is much more aggressive than flossing and considerably more painful.

- Dry needling: Think of this like acupuncture with electrical current (yes, it hurts like hell). Use this when a muscle is seized up.

Again, I don't recommend any of these protocols without a professional.

PUTTING IT ALL TOGETHER

Before we move on to the next section, I wanted to share a few more thoughts about mobility. You should become a student of your body's movement. When you're driving a car that is misaligned, you feel it pull away from the direction you want to drive. If you're having difficulty moving your body, then identify the past injuries or muscle imbalances that may be causing your misdirection. A physical therapist or a personal trainer with experience in corrective exercise can help you identify and heal your imbalances.

Then focus your attention on the issues they identify. Not only is it a waste of time to stretch your entire body, but it can also be counterproductive. Because I sit as much as I do, my buttocks spend a lot of time in a lengthened state. There's no value in stretching them. My calves and hip flexors? You bet!

Make mobility something you work on every day, or at the very least, on most days. When you've pinpointed the parts of yourself that need the work, dedicate time to them. It doesn't have to be much, but five to ten minutes each day can go a long way toward improving mobility.

ENDURANCE

It shouldn't surprise you that my mind is often drawn back to that day in Puerto Vallarta when I had to sub out of the volleyball game.

Ten years earlier, I'd completed a fifty-mile trail run. I had always thought of myself as an endurance athlete. However, my failure to train for endurance caused me to lose that ability, and I lost a piece of myself in the process.

You don't have to go to the extreme with endurance. This

is one of the modalities that you should train only in alignment with your vision. Build up your endurance to suit the lifestyle you want to have—without going overboard—and that will look very different for each of us.

CARDIO AND WEIGHT LIFTING— WHICH COMES FIRST?

One of the most common workout questions people ask me is:

"I want to lift weights and do cardio as part of my fitness routine—which should I do first each day?"

I follow that question with one of my own: Can you do two sessions—one in the morning and another in the afternoon or evening?

If so, I recommend doing cardio training in the morning and resistance training in the afternoon or evening. But if you have to do them in one session, I'd do resistance work first and close out with cardio. Each of these options gives you the maximum energy output for your resistance training.

ENOUGH ENDURANCE TO WALK THE ZOO

I worked with a client named Susan who would get winded walking from her front door to her car in the driveway. I asked Susan to make an addition to her morning routine: instead of just walking directly to her car, she would take a lap around the car. She reported back that it was hard, but she managed to complete her task. A few days later, we upped it to two laps and continued this process until, in a matter of weeks, she was walking around the neighborhood.

Susan's *why* was her granddaughter. Prior to our working together, Susan would be exhausted just playing with her granddaughter for a few hours. She couldn't dream of going to the zoo and keeping up with this bundle of energy running from the giraffes over to the lions and the monkeys. But she wanted to, so she trained her endurance just enough for that goal.

Some people derive major mental and emotional benefits from endurance training. I have one client for whom running contributes significantly to his mental well-being; he has to do a six-mile run at least once a week to feel *normal*. There aren't too many people who would need to run that far as part of their vision, but it makes him happy, which is a part of wellness.

For most of you, you're more like Susan: you have to find the balance that best suits you—the one most aligned to your vision.

THE CYCLE OF GYM LIFE

Every year, during the first week of January, a bunch of new faces show up at the gym with the "deer in the headlights" look. Then they find the closest available treadmill because it seems safe. Then every time they come in after that, they beeline to the same comfortable treadmill and go wherever it takes them, which is nowhere. Three weeks later, they stop showing up because they see no progress—they've lost to their own resolution.

At first, these new gym-goers choose the treadmill for two reasons: it's familiar to them and they want to burn calories to lose weight. As you know, neither of those alone is a good reason to train, but there is a time and place for cardio machines in your training. They can be great tools to help you train for endurance, especially during inclement weather or when you're recovering from an injury, but I'd encourage you to take your endurance training outside as it will make it much more enjoyable.

Training for endurance is relatively simple: slow, incremental pushes (i.e., progression) will get you there.

You don't have to run one mile today, two miles tomorrow, and three miles the next day, and on and on and on. In fact, that's the opposite of how you safely build endurance. If you try to add too much too fast, you'll injure yourself, and at our age, any injury can set us back an incredible amount of time.

In a basic approach I use with my clients, we have a short-distance day, a moderate-distance day, and a long day. After the long day, we have a rest day. For example, they may walk half a mile on Monday, a mile on Tuesday, and two miles on Wednesday, then take Thursday off and pick up the cycle again on Friday. After they've gotten comfortable with this walking program, we can focus on either moving faster or increasing the distance.

If you want to be a runner, I'd recommend Jeff Galloway's Run Walk Run Method™. The method lets you safely build the endurance to become a runner by teaching you how to avoid redlining. When you can train at your endurance threshold, you're able to build up capacity quickly and effectively.

HIGH-INTENSITY INTERVAL TRAINING

You may have heard of high-intensity interval training (HIIT). This training protocol is a supercharged way to build endurance. The biggest advantage for HIIT is the time efficiency. Most HIIT workouts go for less than thirty minutes, with some as short as four minutes. Let me take just a minute to explain how HIIT works.

During a HIIT session, you cycle through an intense workout for a short time (no longer than thirty seconds), followed by a short period of rest.

The intensity in high-intensity interval training means you work at the same intensity you would if you were running from an angry bear with your baby in your arms. You keep up that intensity for the full work period (or else that bear is going to catch you, and, well, it won't be pretty). Then you get a chance to rest (think of a light walk through the woods) until it's time to start the next work period—meaning another bear comes around, and he looks meaner than the first. RUN!

Get the point?

It will wear you out, and because it is such a shock to your metabolic system, you should limit yourself to only one HIIT session every five to seven days.

BALANCE

Every day in the United States, more than one in four adults aged sixty-five and older will sustain a fall.[6] Those falls result in three million emergency room visits, 800,000 hospitalizations, and 28,000 deaths. Falls

---

6   "Important Facts about Falls," Centers for Disease Control and Prevention, https://www.cdc. gov/homeandrecreationalsafety/falls/adultfalls.html.

are the number one cause of injury and injury-induced deaths in older Americans.[7]

Falls are the end for a lot of seniors, so they are right to be afraid. As such, there is an entire industry built around products for seniors who are at risk of falling. When people are afraid to fall, they shorten their walking gait. It's a little-known and seemingly innocent phenomenon, but by shortening their gait, older people are actually creating a smaller base of balance, which makes them even more susceptible to falls.

MY SELF-AWARENESS

Balance is my worst fitness modality. I'm the kind of guy who would fail a field sobriety test even when completely sober. As a result, this modality is becoming much more of a priority for me.

Here's a good test of your balance: stand with both feet relatively close together. How balanced do you feel? Now lift one foot off the ground. Can you hold it up for thirty seconds? What about the other foot? Maybe that was easy for you. What happens when you close your eyes? Even if you're relatively strong in this modality, these tests of your balance could land you face-first on the ground.

---

7   "Falls Are Leading Cause of Injury and Death in Older Americans," Centers for Disease Control and Prevention, https://www.cdc.gov/media/releases/2016/p0922-older-adult-falls.html.

Balance is an issue for many of us, and now you know where that road takes you: falls, broken hips, and a shortened life. But the good news is that balance, like all fitness modalities, can improve through training.

Improving your balance is shockingly simple: put yourself in unbalanced positions and try to maintain them. Even better, pair these unbalanced positions with dynamic movements like single-arm overhead dumbbell presses. That's what balance is all about: being comfortable in an unbalanced state.

ONE WORD OF CAUTION

When you're working on your balance, make sure you're in a space where you won't hurt yourself if you do lose your balance.

SPEED AND AGILITY

One of the first things my high school tennis coach taught me was that I had to arrive at the spot where I wanted to make contact with the ball *before* the ball got there. Well, duh! But really, having the speed to be in the correct position is harder than it sounds. Also, when you're not in the position you need to be in, you're more likely to make a sad swipe at the ball and lose the point.

When you break down the seemingly simple movement

of a tennis swing, you find that it's more complex than you might think: you run to the ball, stop, turn your body, set your feet, and draw the racket back. There are a lot of moving parts. Do you have the speed and agility to pull that off?

Maybe you don't play tennis. Fair enough. Instead, maybe you want to teach your granddaughter hopscotch, or start trail running, or learn to two-step dance. Or maybe you just want to make sure you can avoid a car being operated by a careless driver.

"We don't stop playing because we grow old. We grow old because we stop playing."

—GEORGE BERNARD SHAW

The cool thing about training speed and agility is that it feels more like play than it does work. I can't say that for many of the other fitness modalities. Play should be part of all of our lives. I'm sure I'm not speaking out of turn when I say we all hate being stuck in rush hour traffic. Driving is fun when it involves speed and agility—same with our lives.

One area where most people over forty struggle is with side-to-side movement. We walk forward, we stand up, and we sit down. Everything we do is on a linear plane, which does very little to improve our agility.

You can fix that with simple side-to-side steps as you stand at the sink washing dishes, for example. As you move between the sink and the cupboards, make it a side-to-side shuffle.

As you progress with your agility, you can go into the backyard and turn the sidestepping into dynamic movements. Step side to side with your left foot, then bring you right foot to meet it, do another step left, then repeat the sequence back to the right. Once that movement becomes too easy, you can cross your feet as you step: right foot over your left foot, left foot out, right foot behind your left foot, left foot out, and so on. That's called a carioca exercise, and once you get the hang of it, it can be very fun and it will improve your agility.

SO MUCH TO DO, SO LITTLE TIME

There is value in improving each of these fitness modalities, but improving all of them requires a significant time investment. Is there a way to train all of them at the same time? Yes, there is: it's called cross-training. Some boot-camp-style classes will incorporate most, if not all, of the modalities we've covered, but I've found that focusing on two or three often nets much better results.

So we have to prioritize the work we do based on the time we have. We have different baggage and passengers on our wellness journey. Remember? We have to ask ourselves three questions:

- Based on the pace I've set for myself, how much time can I devote to training?
- Which fitness modalities will move me further down the road toward my vision?
- What are my nonnegotiables?

Time is a limited resource. Because you're committed to your wellness goal, you're going to make sure you allocate time to train. In a general sense, you must commit to training at least three hours per week, although it would be optimal if you could train for seven hours per week. And before you freak out, thinking you could never make that commitment, seven hours per week is probably less time than you spend watching TV. It represents about 4 percent of the 168 hours you have in a week. That's doable for most of us—if you're committed.

There is another significance to exercising seven hours per week: if you work for one hour a day, you're meeting your seven-hour goal *and* you're doing something for your fitness every day. That's how habits are born.

Make fitness a habit.

Which modalities are necessary to reach your vision? I'd

be willing to put money on body composition (what other people call weight loss) as being either number one or number two on your list of modalities aligned to your vision. However, that's my guess; you'll have to spend time thinking through your roadmap to discover what will move the needle most for you.

For me, the most important modality is strength. Yours might be endurance to keep up with grandbabies or mobility because you're struggling with back issues.

Ask yourself: *What is the one fitness modality that you can't live without maintaining?*

This is your nonnegotiable. Even though the client I mentioned earlier doesn't need a high level of endurance to reach his vision, it is his nonnegotiable because it brings him peace.

Once you have your modalities prioritized, you have direction. From there, you can begin learning what training you'll want to do in order to achieve results for each specific modality. As you work your way through the STREETS on your wellness roadmap, you'll learn how to get maximum return for the time and effort you invest.

But wait, what is that I see on the horizon—a rest stop? On this journey you're taking, you can't just drive and drive and drive without stopping; you need to rest, too. Let's learn more about this magical place called the rest stop, where sleep and recovery actually make your trip go faster.

CHAPTER 6

REST

On January 28, 1986, I saw my future career—the reason I was in college majoring in physics—die with the *Challenger* space shuttle. As I watched the news stations replay the footage of the shuttle disintegrating into a million pieces, one thought stuck in my head: *There was a civilian on that mission, and they just died. NASA won't fly another shuttle until they find every piece of that aircraft, find out what happened, and figure out how to make sure it never happens again.*

I dreamed of a space program where shuttles would be like airlines, flying up and down to the International Space Station, bringing people and supplies between space and Earth. My dream of going to space shattered in that moment when the shuttle exploded.

I'd reached a pivot point: either continue in school for a

major I didn't enjoy for an outcome that was no longer possible, or make a change. So rather than continuing to pay for school, I joined the Army as an infantry soldier. It gave me an opportunity to get back to my athletic days and get a paycheck instead of paying tuition.

Light infantry soldiers are the elite athletes of the military—we had to carry our equipment and ourselves everywhere we went. Nobody could carry that load without some serious physical fitness. I was already a very good runner with a high endurance level when I enlisted, so basic training came easily for me. It was kind of boring, actually.

I'm a competitor; I'm always looking for my next challenge. When I saw that my training unit was forming a team for a base-wide running competition, I signed up immediately and got to work.

Just like you'd see in the movies, our team of twenty soldiers ran around in line formations, our chants echoing across the base while our drill sergeant ran alongside us making cadence calls. Our training regimen was much more intense than the normal basic training: we ran farther and faster than everyone not in the competition. And I loved every minute of it.

Until my body started breaking down.

The problem was that the military—at the time—didn't understand the importance of rest. Even as a hotshot twenty-year-old, I knew I needed a day to recover after a hard run, but we never got a single day off during competition training. We woke up, we ran, we went through the day's physically demanding basic training, we went to bed, and did it all over again the next morning, every single day of the week leading up to our race.

In our drill sergeant's mind, more running meant we had more training in a shorter time, and we would therefore be better come race time. To my twenty-year-old brain, the logic *seemed* sound—more must be better, right? But unfortunately not.

With exercise, if you don't allow yourself time to recover and rebuild, your body will break down. That's exactly what happened to me. About a week before the race, I felt an ache in my groin. It didn't keep me from running, so I continued our regimen. Then, just days before our race date, I felt an agonizing, sharp, shooting pain in my right knee. I was as fit as could be at this point in my life. I had a seemingly endless endurance, and I was very strong. But because of the way my drill sergeant had trained me, my twenty-year-old body was breaking down.

Race day arrived. I knew I was in trouble when we started the warm-up before the race. Here I thought we'd stretch our legs for a light mile for the five-mile race, just to get the blood flowing. I fell into formation and tried to find a groove, hoping to somehow grind this day out. But every step was agony. I could feel the pain shooting up from my knee with every step, jolting through my leg and into my pulled groin.

We reached the mile point and the drill sergeant kept running us. *This is still the warm-up?* He kept upping the pace, too. The weeks-long accumulation of nonstop training with no rest tore me at the seams. The drill sergeant ran us right up until the start of the race. The Army's "hurry up and wait" approach to most things turned into "hurry up and run": we covered seven miles before the race even started.

My blood was pumping, all right—I could feel every pulse throbbing in my knee, accompanied by a deep ache in my groin.

By the time the race started, I had already given everything my body had left and more. But being an athlete and a natural competitor, I refused to give up. *I have to do this*, I told myself. *I have to stay in formation*. If we lost more than two runners from our twenty-man team, we were disqualified. I pushed my body as far as it would go, but there was nothing left to give. I was one of two to fall out. Our team got to the finish, but all I felt was the disappointment and embarrassment of letting them down.

The groin injury was a pull that healed with a few days of rest. But my knee was in really bad shape. The pain in my knee was sharp and shooting. I was terrified that it would keep me from completing training and I'd have to repeat the entire thirteen-week infantry training.

Because of the amount of time I had trained without rest, the tendons and ligaments in my knee became severely damaged and inflamed. They weren't completely torn, because I hadn't done anything overly athletic like twisting and turning—the kinds of motions that would lead to a tear—but they were beaten up to the point that they were just wasted, like rubber bands with no elasticity.

In a scenario like this, where your body senses something wrong, it sends white blood cells in a surge to aid in healing. This causes swelling, which leads to pain. The groin injury was just a strained muscle, which, with good blood flow, was able to heal quickly. However, tendons and ligaments, like the ones in my knee, don't get nearly as much blood flow, so it takes them longer to get those white blood cells to repair.

It took years for my knee to fully recover from that period of intense training with inadequate rest.

Looking back on that race, with the experience I have now as a personal trainer, I can easily see what went wrong. If I'd been given just three or four days of rest, I could have healed my groin. And with the adequate rest, I probably wouldn't have injured my knee. Because our drill sergeant didn't understand the importance of rest and recovery, I never got that time.

REST AND RECOVERY

It's important to understand the concept of rest as it applies to two areas of training: (1) rest between sets and (2) rest between training sessions (otherwise known as recovery). By getting proper rest between sets within a workout, you ensure that you can continue doing the work in the gym to stimulate muscle growth. By getting proper rest outside the gym—between training sessions— you ensure your body has time to fully recover from your training.

Whether you enjoy training or not, to make the most of your time and effort, learn how to rest and recover.

REST BETWEEN SETS

Most prescribed training plans will allow for a period of work followed by a period of rest. I'll be discussing rest from the perspective of resistance training (including strength, muscle mass, and bone density), but rest between sets also applies to other fitness modalities.

By utilizing appropriate rest between sets, you'll optimize your training time and get the most out of your workout.

Taking a rest between sets during a training session allows your muscles to reset. During rest, your muscle flushes out chemical waste by-products and restores its energy cycle. The muscle won't *completely reset* during your rest between sets, which is why the second and third sets are harder than the first, but it should allow you to continue to train hard. The key with rest between sets is to take enough time so your body can get back to an optimal state of performance but not so long that your muscles cool off. For most people, this will be somewhere between 60 and 120 seconds.

For example, if my resistance training session includes three sets of ten back squats, I'll do my first set of ten back squats—where I squat down until my thighs are just past parallel with the ground and press back up—then, once I finish those ten squats, I'll take a sixty-second break before doing ten more. Then I'll take another sixty-second break and do my final set of ten.

That's what works for me, but experiment with what amount of time works for you. As you lift heavier weights, you'll need more time between sets to recover—sometimes as much as three minutes. If you're doing more repetitions at a lighter weight, you can cut back on your rest time between sets.

The Downfalls of Too Much Rest between Sets

We all have a very important, limited, and nonrenewable resource in our lives: **our time.** If you enjoy being in the gym and want to chat with people for five minutes between sets, just be sure you're aware of what you're doing: you're socializing, not training. I don't mean that in a bad way—for some people, the gym is a great social scene. But if you're looking to do what's best for your overall fitness in the least amount of time necessary, then taking too much time between sets is simply a waste of your time.

Additionally, by chatting between sets you're allowing your muscles to cool down. For a younger person, cooling down is not much of a problem. Not so for people over forty. We do warm-ups for a reason: we don't want to injure ourselves. By taking long breaks between sets, you allow your muscles to cool down and you put yourself at risk of injury.

REST BETWEEN TRAINING SESSIONS

Training your body is actually a process of intentionally stressing it in hopes that it will adapt to the load you place on it. That adaptation takes time. Giving your body enough time to recover and rebuild is the key to seeing results from your work.

Push hard when you train, then take the time your body needs to recover.

The time it takes muscles to recover varies from person to person and from muscle to muscle. For example, my leg muscles take longer to recover than my upper-body muscles. You may recover very quickly, but I can tell you this: nobody's recovery time is zero, and I learned that painful lesson the hard way in the military.

You might be able to run seven days a week, but even if you're in peak health, you will, at the very least, need a lighter day thrown in here and there. That's effectively rest and recovery time. Even so, I'd still encourage you to take time off occasionally to let your body fully recover from the work you're putting it through.

After forty, most of us don't recover as quickly as we used to. If you do a great leg-training session with squats, lunges, and some machine work, you might need a full *week* for your legs to recover. That's completely normal, especially when you're just getting started—we older cars aren't as durable or as efficient as the newer models.

As a general rule, you need at least forty-eight hours of recovery time between training sessions for the same muscles. If you work out a muscle group especially hard, you may need as much as seventy-two hours to recover.

As you get older, you'll recover more slowly. When I was in my twenties, forty-eight hours between leg training was plenty of time. Now my recovery time has lengthened, so I give myself at least seventy-two hours. It's a matter of finding what works best for you.

Active Recovery

Active recovery means you keep moving your muscles during the days following your training, but you're not pushing yourself to the same extent you normally do. You're basically moving through a range of motion without resistance, which allows you to get blood flow through your muscles, ligaments, and tendons and helps speed up the recovery process.

Always err on the side of active (as opposed to passive) recovery. I mentioned leg day: if you go hard on your workout, especially with your legs, you'll likely experience delayed onset muscle soreness (remember my Insanity workout?). DOMS isn't a bad thing or a good thing; it just means you've pushed your body to a point that it wasn't quite prepared for. Active rest is the best prescription for DOMS and any similar workout-related muscle soreness.

REPEATED CYCLES: THE DOWNFALLS OF CIRCUIT TRAINING

Most commercial gyms have an area set up for circuit training, where people can efficiently move from machine to machine with as little rest as possible. A circuit might look like this: you do a set of lat pull downs, pulling a bar from overhead down to your chest; you move to the leg extension machine to complete a set; then you get on the chest press machine for a set, and so on through the other machines. Once you finish this circuit, you will have worked all the major muscles in your body.

Most circuit training sessions have you go through all of the exercises two, maybe three times. You may rest between circuits but not between exercises in the circuit. While you're not resting between *sets*, you are working out different sets of muscles back-to-back, so the reset isn't necessary to continue exerting maximum effort.

Circuit training can be a fun and efficient way to build strength, especially if you have a trainer and a group of people to run through the circuits with you. It gives you a full-body workout in half the time of a regular full-body resistance training session.

However, I often see people fall into a pattern with circuit training: they arrive at the gym on Monday and do a circuit. On Tuesday they do the same circuit. Then it's the same story again on Wednesday, Thursday, and Friday. They know their weight settings for each exercise and never change any of them.

Despite the sweating, these individuals don't get stronger—they only stagnate.

The same thing happens with the people on treadmills and elliptical machines: they come in five days a week and do the same thing all five days. Now don't get me wrong: I don't want to pooh-pooh any kind of work—I'm happy when anyone is at the gym—but you could progress a lot faster if you took the time to understand that your muscles need rest in order to build.

If you can go into the gym the very next day and execute the same workout with the same weight, then you didn't push yourself hard enough the day before. A good strength training session—one with adequate resistance—makes you want a day of rest.

THE DEFINITION OF INSANITY?

Albert Einstein said, "The definition of insanity is doing the same thing over and over again and expecting a different result." Einstein himself was never sure he really said that quote, and no one could point to a specific time he said it, but he did agree that it was sage advice.

Your goal should be to increase your strength, not maintain it. Sarcopenia sets in as you age, and your body requires more intensity and more recovery in order to stave off that 1 percent loss of muscle mass every year.

As a teenager, I had a job unloading trucks. The boxes all weighed sixty pounds. I went on the truck, grabbed a box, carried it down a ramp, and stacked it in the warehouse. Every day, I hauled the same type of boxes, all exactly the same weight. Once my body got comfortable with the sixty-pound boxes, I could unload them all day—I was comfortable at that weight and work output. But I made no progress: my strength and endurance stagnated. In order to progress, I needed to lift heavier boxes.

You have to push yourself in order to progress. Circuits that you repeat every day at the same weights don't lead to progress, and without progress, you'll feel frustrated as you put in work for no improvement on results.

SLEEP

Have you ever seen a mechanic work on a car's engine while it was running? Hopefully, your answer is a resounding no.

Now, your mechanic may turn your car on to diagnose a problem, but while they do the repairs, the engine is certainly off. Otherwise, they risk serious injury. For our bodies, sleep is when we effectively turn off our engine and allow our bodies to repair and restore themselves.

We must sleep, whether we want to or not. While even the experts aren't sure exactly why we evolved to require sleep, it's clear that it significantly impacts our health. Yes, the amount of sleep we get matters immensely—the general consensus is that we need between six to nine hours per night—but sleep quality matters just as much.

THE SLEEP CYCLE

High-quality sleep means you get an unencumbered chance for your body to work through all four sleep stages: shallow sleep, intermediate sleep, deep sleep, and rapid eye movement (REM) sleep. A normal sleep cycle, one in which you go through all four stages, lasts ninety minutes for most people. A complete sleep cycle with all four stages ensures that you're giving your brain what it needs to function well.

FOUR OR FIVE?

Some experts break deep sleep into two categories: deep sleep and *very* deep sleep, which results in five sleep stages. For simplicity, we'll stick with the four stages model in this book.

Deep sleep is important because it shuts the body down, and your brain begins producing delta waves. Experts believe this is the time when your brain cleanses itself. REM sleep is the period of the sleep cycle when we dream. Experts believe this is when we manage the storage of memory.

Through extensive experimentation with apps and devices, I've discovered that I need four or five good sleep cycles each night to wake up refreshed. In order to get good, refreshing sleep, you should avoid being woken up in deep sleep or REM sleep. That's why I go to bed early enough that I don't need to set an alarm to wake me up, and I wake up naturally when I'm in a light sleep cycle. As a result, I wake feeling well-rested.

You can buy apps to track your sleep or buy an alarm that

monitors your sleep cycle and wakes you during light sleep, but I find that simply recording when you go to bed, when you wake up, and how you feel in the morning lets you learn how to optimize your bedtime. (We'll talk more about journaling and bedtimes later in this chapter.)

HORMONES AND SLEEP

Good hormone balance is critical to our wellness. There is a direct interaction between our sleep and many of our key hormones: both follow the circadian rhythm. A circadian rhythm is how the twenty-four-hour cycle (day and night) affects our bodies. When we go against the normal day/night process, such as working night shifts, our health suffers.

Living on a schedule that takes you off the natural circadian rhythm results in unfavorable hormone production. Hormones are like messengers in our bodies—they tell our bodies what to do and how to do it.

When I turn the key in my car's ignition, it sends a signal— much like hormones—for the starter to fire up the engine. If you don't have the right key for the car, your car won't start. If your hormones aren't balanced, you're not going to function well, and wellness in all its forms will be out of your reach.

There are several hormones that are affected by and affect your sleep, including:

- Thyroid
- Testosterone, estrogen, and progesterone
- Insulin
- Cortisol

THYROID

Your thyroid regulates the thyroid hormones, which tell your body how much energy you need. Poor thyroid function can cause night sweats, which disrupt your sleep, and it can also cause weight gain, which can result in sleep apnea. Thyroid health can be improved through proper nutrition. If you're having issues with your energy levels and sleep quality, it's worth having your thyroid levels tested.

SLEEP APNEA

Sleep apnea is a condition where we stop breathing during sleep. As you might imagine, it makes it hard to complete a full sleep cycle. As with snoring in general, the core recommendation for sleep apnea treatment is to lose weight. But if you're showing symptoms of sleep apnea (your spouse may notice moments when you've stopped breathing completely), get a sleep study done to determine if you have it. Get the help you need because poor sleep causes weight gain and weight gain only makes sleep apnea worse.

TESTOSTERONE, ESTROGEN, AND PROGESTERONE

These three hormones are known as the sex hormones. If we aren't in good balance with our sex hormones, we'll never get to true wellness. Insomnia is a common symptom of sex hormones being out of whack.

Testosterone is necessary for muscle growth. Our testosterone naturally peaks in the early morning. Of course, that's why men feel a bit more—ahem—*amorous* when we first wake up. Poor sleep quality can disrupt testosterone synthesis. Good sleep, therefore, results in better muscle building from your resistance training.

Women also experience issues when their estrogen and progesterone aren't balanced, such as hot flashes and night sweats. Menopause especially wreaks havoc on the estrogen/progesterone balance.

INSULIN

Insulin is a very important hormone that regulates blood sugar. If you're prediabetic or diabetic, your kidneys work to rid your blood of excess sugar through the urine. This can cause you to get up several times throughout the night to pee. The double whammy is that sleep deprivation can induce insulin resistance. It's a vicious circle.

CORTISOL

Cortisol is the stress hormone. It naturally spikes in the morning to help us wake up. This hormone also triggers a fight-or-flight response in the body. Staying in a high cortisol state is bad for two reasons: it is catabolic—meaning it breaks down muscle—and it can disrupt sleep.

All of these hormones function in our bodies to help us look, feel, and be well. To build muscle, you want your testosterone at the right level. Cortisol, on the other hand, is catabolic and will keep you from gaining muscle if it isn't kept in check. Insulin is the hormone that most affects weight gain or loss. And the thyroid controls our energy. Sleep affects all of these hormones and all of these hormones in turn affect our sleep.

I have my hormone levels checked each time I go to the doctor for a wellness visit. You may not need to check yours that often, but it is worth getting a baseline for your hormone production. Then you can start tracking how nutrition, exercise, and sleep can optimize your hormone balance, which will help you along your journey to wellness.

SLEEP HYGIENE

Good sleep should be a major priority in your life. For most people, this is an obvious, but potentially life-changing, mindset change. Good sleep is like getting a tune-up for your car: it's a ritual of renewal and replenishment that keeps you on the road to wellness.

Sleep hygiene gives you the best chance of getting good sleep. The elements of good sleep hygiene are:

- Having a consistent bedtime
- Managing light exposure
- Performing a sleep ritual
- Creating a good sleep environment
- Avoiding sleep disruptors

HAVING A CONSISTENT BEDTIME

In his book *The Power of When*, Dr. Michael Breus identifies four chronotypes: dolphin, lion, bear, and wolf. These chronotypes provide insight over the optimal time for you to sleep.

I'm a lion, meaning I want to get up early and attack the day. My bedtime is 8:30 p.m., which most people think is insane, but I wake up at 3:30 a.m. or 4:00 a.m., having completed all of my sleep cycles. By waking up so early, I have about three or four hours in the morning when nobody's emailing me and I can get my work done.

Bears, the most common chronotype, follow the schedule

of the sun. Wolves stay up late at night and like to sleep in. And dolphins may or may not have a regular sleep pattern.

Regardless of your chronotype, the most important thing you can do to improve your sleep hygiene is creating a consistent bedtime. You can learn more about the chronotypes by visiting thepowerofwhenquiz.com.

MANAGING LIGHT EXPOSURE

Televisions, computer screens, and phones emit blue light, much like the sky does during the day. But as the sun goes down, you'll notice more oranges and reds in the sky. Our bodies have adapted to that color change: blue tells us to stay awake, reds and oranges tell us to go to bed.

Apps such as f.lux filter out the blue light on computer screens as we drift into evening time, and most phones have the technology to do the same. Even so, using an app is not a fix-all. I know it's hard to put down the phone in the middle of a Words with Friends game or to stop bingeing on Netflix, but these habits stimulate your mind in the evenings, making it harder for you to get to sleep.

Get away from all screens at least a half hour before bedtime. That will give you enough time to incorporate the next sleep hygiene element.

PERFORMING A BEDTIME RITUAL

Rituals teach our bodies how we need them to respond. I'm fairly certain that you brush and floss before bed (I hope). Taking care of our dental hygiene before bed is a ritual we've been doing all our lives. It's a key signal to the body that it's time to sleep. The only problem is that the brain doesn't always get that signal. Sometimes it wants to turn on just as we want it to turn off.

There are some additional rituals you can adopt in order to teach your mind that it's time to go to bed.

Light a candle (which emits the orange light of natural evening time) and do some journaling. This journal can be where you dump the feelings and thoughts that stress you out. It can also be a place for you to get organized for the next day by creating a to-do list. I also encourage you to use it as a gratitude journal. Gratitude is a very powerful emotion that not only helps you relax for a more restful sleep, but it also allows you to let go of the day.

I also enjoy reading fiction before bed. Some people use this time before bed to meditate. Whatever works for you. The point is to wind down and communicate to your body that it is time to sleep. Sleep rituals create a natural boundary between your day and your night. As you build this nightly ritual, your mind and body will do a better job of winding down and turning off.

CREATING A GOOD SLEEP ENVIRONMENT

Long before I knew about the issues with blue light, I made the decision that I would never have a television in my bedroom, and that decision has really served me well. Your bedroom should serve only two purposes: sleep and—well, you know. It should be a special place where no other activities outside of those two are allowed.

I also make our bedroom as dark as possible. I use blackout shades, and we don't have any nightlights in the room. I don't even take my phone into the bedroom (my wife does, but she's kind enough to go into the other room if she feels the need to use it). We have a very low nightlight in the bathroom that is motion activated. Otherwise, I can get back and forth between the bedroom and the bathroom and only *occasionally* step on a dog along the way.

You'll also get better sleep if you keep your bedroom cool. I prefer it at sixty-five degrees or cooler, but my wife likes it warmer, so we compromise with sixty-eight to seventy. If she's not around, though, I'm cranking it all the way down to sixty-three. Of course, you'll want to experiment with what feels most comfortable for you (and your spouse).

You'll also want to address noise as a part of your sleep environment. If you live in a city, you might be comfortable with street noise. I prefer white noise, so I run a fan at night. You may also want to use earplugs if you need absolute silence to sleep.

Finally, make sure your bedding helps facilitate good sleep. Invest in a good mattress and pillows. When you have good bedding, you'll be more comfortable and you won't toss and turn in the night. You should wake up feeling rested and refreshed, not achy, sore, and exhausted.

Make your bedroom a Fortress of Solitude—quiet, dark, and cool with comfortable bedding. You'll sleep better for it.

TO NAP OR NOT TO NAP

You may have heard that naps are bad, but I beg to differ. I love naps, so long as I get in a full sleep cycle. My napping habits go against the conventional wisdom that encourages short power naps, but I've never felt better after a short nap. I also won't nap after 4:00 p.m. Other than those two rules, if I'm feeling sleepy and I have the time, I'll gladly go into a ninety-minute snooze. That's what works best for me. Experiment to find what works best for you.

AVOIDING SLEEP DISRUPTORS

Avoid eating right before bed. I know it's so tempting to have some munchies while you watch Netflix, but eating before bed forces your digestive system to keep working after it's time to turn off. Also, raising your blood sugar can impair sleep.

A lot of people use alcohol or prescription drugs to fall asleep. My response to those habits is simple: just don't. You may fall asleep faster on pills and alcohol, but you won't get good sleep. Alcohol and most sleep aids don't allow us to properly complete sleep cycles. Focus instead on the other elements of good sleep hygiene to get your body to sleep.

As you get better sleep, you notice your hormone production improves, which makes you feel better. You look better, you move more, and you balance your hormones. Suddenly, you're on a powerful upward spiral.

We're all busy people. We think working hard on little rest is a sign of status and importance. In reality, sleep is the best way to make sure you benefit from the work you're doing, not only in physical wellness but also in emotional and mental wellness. Spending hours working out and eating right won't get you far if you don't rest and recover. Rest is where you make some of the best time on your wellness journey.

HOW I REPAIRED THIS OLD PICKUP TRUCK

I was injured when I begrudgingly dropped out of that race in basic training, but I was still in incredible shape in terms of endurance and cardiovascular health.

As we continued with basic training, we prepared for

the Army Physical Training (PT) test, which included a two-mile run. After all the work I'd put in, training for a two-mile run was nothing but active recovery.

Within days, my groin healed, but my knee was just starting the healing process. By the time the PT test came up, the inflammation had gone away and I was able to complete the two-mile run at a time I was very happy with.

I was in my twenties, so recovery came relatively quickly. At fifty-two, it takes me much longer to recover. I train smarter and I listen to my body and give it the rest and recovery it needs. You have to take care of the body you have; it's the only one you've got.

Your recovery is dependent on maintaining your body—or your vehicle—by doing things such as getting regular oil changes, which means resting and sleeping on a consistent basis. I currently drive a 2010 Ford pickup truck with more than 265,000 miles on it. Because I get regular oil changes and I don't push it too hard, it runs as well as it did the day I bought it new. Get the rest and sleep your body needs, and it will serve you well.

CHAPTER 7

——

ENERGY

Other than the speedometer, the gas gauge is where your eyes go to the most on your dashboard. You can't get anywhere without enough of the right kind of fuel. Likewise, your wellness won't improve without the right kind of nutrition. Sometimes finding the right fuel takes a little experimentation.

I call this chapter Energy because I'm covering nutrition. However, I want you to understand that food is so much more than just fuel. It gives us the energy to be ourselves and the materials to build ourselves, and it is an integral part of the events that make us who we are. As you may already know, the most important parts of our lives are the parts that are hardest to change. Changing your energy will move you forward on the road to wellness the most.

Every doctor I've ever had believes I'm about to immediately drop dead of a heart attack because I have extremely high cholesterol numbers. The normal range for LDL cholesterol is around 170—mine usually ebbs and flows between 250 and 300. That said, my total cholesterol-to-HDL ratio is better than the recommended level, and my triglycerides are well below the 150 range that most doctors believe is healthy.

Cholesterol serves as a building block for many important hormones. We've already discussed hormones as they relate to sleep, but I have to reemphasize this point: you will never look, feel, or be well if you don't have good hormone balance.

I believe medical professionals obsess over high cholesterol way too much. I've never seen a study that definitively ties high cholesterol with early mortality. In fact, of the people who have heart attacks, 75 percent have normal cholesterol levels.[8]

8   Rachel Champeau, "Most Heart Attack Patients' Cholesterol Levels Did Not Indicate Cardiac Risk," UCLA News Room, January 12, 2009, http://newsroom.ucla.edu/releases/majority-of-hospitalized-heart-75668.

CHOLESTEROL: THE JURY IS STILL OUT

In my opinion, the jury is still out on cholesterol. I've seen studies that show an inverse relationship between total and LDL cholesterol and all causes of mortality. In effect, some studies conclude that the lower your cholesterol is, the more likely you're going to die, especially from cancer and heart disease. Still, many doctors insist that higher cholesterol is bad for us, and put us on meds to lower those levels.

In short, the conventional wisdom states that you should lower your cholesterol, but more studies are showing that lower cholesterol is actually bad for you. So, in my opinion, the jury's still out.

I go to the doctor for wellness visits three to four times a year. Every time we talk, like déjà vu, his eyes light up and he says, "Oh wow! Would you look at those cholesterol numbers. We better get you on some medication." The few times I relented and tried statins and niacin, the side effects were horrible.

Having read *Cholesterol Clarity* by Jimmy Moore and Dr. Eric Westman, I found myself in a cholesterol tug-of-war with my doctor. Jimmy and Dr. Westman presented a very compelling case against the current standard of care for high cholesterol. My doctor wanted me to cycle through the various medications until I found one I could tolerate. But I've never wanted a *tolerable* existence—I want an optimal life.

Still, it was really hard to go through those quarterly talks. I'd get chastised by my doctor and argue with him about the cholesterol-lowering drugs. After one of our cholesterol sessions, I decided to try something different: I'd fix the problem with nutrition.

I'd recently interviewed a few authors of vegetarian and vegan nutrition books: Dr. Michael Greger, author of *How Not to Die*, and Dr. Thomas Campbell, author of *The China Study Solution*. Both of them had stressed that a primarily plant-based lifestyle would prolong life and have amazing effects on cholesterol. I decided to try it their way—sort of.

HOW I ACTUALLY GAINED WEIGHT EATING PESCATARIAN

I knew I wouldn't be able to play the game of "tofu and bean-based meat substitutes" on my nutrition plan. While there are vegan and vegetarian bodybuilders, I was not willing to jump through so many hoops to get the protein needed to build and maintain muscle mass. So I decided to go pescatarian. I allowed myself to eat up to two servings of fish or shellfish every day. Beyond that, I was full-on vegetarian.

I followed this protocol for three months. My LDL cholesterol went from 305 to 274, which is still more than 100 points above the recommended level of 170. Likewise, my HDL plummeted, down from 89 to 49 (health guidance suggests your HDL stay above 50). My triglyceride levels remained steady. Basically, I was in worse cardiovascular health than when I started.

I also gained ten pounds.

You might wonder how that's possible when all I was eating was vegetables, fruits, nuts, and fish. I know when I pictured vegetarians, I envisioned little thin guys with small arms. Here's the difference with me: most of those skinny vegetarians aren't lifting heavy weights. With all of my energy expenditures in the weight room and my endurance training, I was hungry all the time, and the only things that seemed to fill me up were nuts and fruit.

I was not satiated throughout the day, so I grazed constantly. I had food on my desk, food in my truck—pretty much anytime I wasn't sleeping, showering, or brushing my teeth, I was eating.

There are a lot of people for whom grazing is a great method of getting their nutritional energy. For me, it wasn't. That's what this all comes down to: you have to choose what works for *you* and your lifestyle. Find that balance between lifestyle and the health markers you believe in to get wellness. If there were just one way to get to wellness, there wouldn't be thousands of books about nutrition.

I'm one of the weird people who actually became less healthy eating vegetarian. I know it was a function of my food choices, but a grazing lifestyle doesn't give me the control I need. Maybe you're one of the people who can succeed by grazing all day. All of our engines are different; take the time to find the right fuel for your vehicle.

STUCK IN THE MUD

I'd like to share a story that perfectly contrasts with my pescatarian experience. I'd just returned to a low-carb high-fat (LCHF) way of eating. I woke up early one morning and went out to do some work on a piece of property I own. As I finished up after a few hours, my truck got stuck in the mud.

I called AAA to get towed out. An hour later, the tow truck arrived, only to break down itself as it tried to pull me out. Three hours later, the driver had fixed his truck and I was finally free from the mud. I'd spent those hours fishing (that's why I'd bought the land).

I was driving home and it occurred to me that I hadn't eaten in more than twenty hours. While I'd spent much of the day fishing, I had also done some hard work—all without eating.

There is no way I could have done that as a low-fat pescatarian. My body was now comfortable tapping into my fat to get the reserve energy it needed. It was really nice to have the freedom to do what I needed without being obsessed about my next meal.

SEASONAL KETOSIS

I did a 23andMe DNA test and discovered that my ancestors came from Northern and Eastern Europe. Yes, I'm 100 percent a white guy. There aren't any tropical fruits in that part of the world, and the fruits they did have were very seasonal. Fruit would only grow in the spring and summer, meaning everyone had a short time window to get berries, apples, nuts, and so on. My ancestors would then feast on those carbohydrates and simple sugars while they could.

I believe humans are naturally inclined to be opportunistic eaters. When berries were in season, my ancestors ate all the berries they could. But berries are only available for a short time before they're gone. When plants were scarce during the winter, it was fish, fowl, and small mammals they'd go for. They're harder to catch and kill than a plant, but there is little risk of injury hunting critters and fishing. It would have been rare for them to hunt for bear or elk (much riskier prey), but they would have if the need was great enough.

We still eat opportunistically—it just looks a little different today. It's easier to use the drive-through at a fast food place than it is to shop for good food and prepare it at home. Also, when you have unhealthy snacks in the cupboard, how likely are you to binge? You can't help yourself—it's just how most of us are wired. Our opportunistic eating was necessary for our ancestors' survival, but it is a detriment in our time of abundant food.

> ## LOOK AT ME!
>
> Be wary of doctors who tout their own meal plans and their plans only. They may be so attached to their opinions that they've forgotten to investigate the science backing them up or to look for science that might go against their approach. They suffer from a confirmation bias: they only look for information that supports what they already believe. Don't fall for them, and also be aware of any confirmation bias you might have.

My blood sugar skyrocketed and I gained weight after eating all the tropical fruit—like bananas, pineapples, and oranges—because I'm not built for it. After looking at my eating style and my genetic history, I decided to start seasonal ketosis.

Most of us eating the standard American diet (SAD) are what we call sugar burners: we eat food that contains simple or complex carbohydrates, which our body converts into glucose, and then we burn that glucose for energy. We either use it up through movement and body functions, or it's stored as fat.

An alternate source of energy in our bodies is ketones, which come from fat. To put yourself into ketosis, you eat a very low carbohydrate diet. Most of your calories in ketosis will come from fat—either the fat you eat or the fat on your body. (Remember that day my truck was stuck in the mud? I was in ketosis at the time, so my body was living off my own fat reserves.) When your body has limited access to glucose for energy, it switches to burning fat stores to create the energy you need. That's one of the primary reasons we have body fat (that and to keep us warm in cold weather).

So you can be a sugar burner or a fat burner—but I have to stress the *or*. When your body has adequate glucose, it won't *need* to burn fat. One of the reasons we get fat is that when we eat a diet with lots of carbs and fat, it loads us up with calories. I don't think counting calories is the answer, but realize that both vegan and ketogenic diets can lead to weight loss. You just have to find the one that works best for you. (I'm in the keto camp for most of the year.)

KETOGENIC

To get into ketosis, you have to manage your carbo-hydrates. The standard ratio in calories is as follows:

65 to 75 percent fats

20 to 25 percent proteins (closer to 25 if you're lifting weights consistently)

5 percent carbohydrates

To simplify things, most people will get into ketosis if they're eating twenty grams of carbs or less. Depending on your activity level, genetics, and insulin sensitivity, you may be able to eat more carbs than that and stay in ketosis. In either case, make the carbs you eat count by getting them from locally sourced, organic vegetables.

Seasonal ketosis simply means I choose one season to feast in (like my ancestors) and I'm more diligent about my nutrition the rest of the year. Because I love tailgating for college football season (go Southern Miss!) and I enjoy Thanksgiving, Christmas, and celebrating New Year's Eve with my friends and family, I choose the fall as my feast season. I still try to stay *reasonably* clean with the food I choose, but I do want to enjoy what I eat (I love beer, so I don't worry much about carbs during my feasting season). After the feast season, I go into a famine mode, during which I eat very low carb and I focus more on high-quality proteins and good fats.

The ketogenic diet was developed as an aid to prevent

epileptic seizures,[9] and now scientists are researching it as a potential means of slowing the progress of certain cancers. Many cancers cannot burn ketones for energy—they *require* glucose. So if you restrict the glucose in your body, you could restrict the growth of a tumor. But I must say that this research is all in progress, so no conclusions can be drawn—more studies on the effect of the ketogenic diet on cancer are needed.

In general, I gain about ten to fifteen pounds during the fall, then once I start the famine period I shed that weight, and by summertime, I've leaned up. During my famine period, I keep my carbs below twenty grams per day and gradually lower my total calories and increase my activity level. The result is fat loss. And if I'm lifting heavy, I typically gain some muscle.

There are some people who think eating a high-fat diet will clog your arteries (I don't). You'll want to confer with your doctor before you start any nutrition plan. When you make a significant nutritional change, it can affect the medications you take. (We'll talk more about finding out what works for you in chapter 8, Education.)

When my adoptive father died, I inherited his GMC truck, which had two gas tanks. He needed that because he lived

9   "Ketogenic Diet," Epilepsy Society, https://www.epilepsysociety.org.uk/ketogenic-diet#. WtRuNNPwbow.

in the Utah desert, where there can be more than one hundred miles between gas stations. When I drove down the road and switched tanks, there was always a little sputter as the engine switched from one energy source to another. There's a little hiccup. That's what happens when you shift from being a sugar (glucose) burner to a fat (ketone) burner. It can be very difficult to change from being a sugar burner to a fat burner—some people even get what's called the keto flu when they start.

It is this period that makes some people think that the ketogenic diet is unsustainable. But once you push through the keto flu and get adapted to being a fat burner, you'll feel wonderful and have tons of energy.

Ketosis works for me; it feels great and the food tastes delicious! I do go through the dip each time I come out of my feasting season, but I'm finding it easier and easier to make the switch as time goes on. I believe I'm much more metabolically flexible now than when I was just a sugar burner.

Because I'm not insulin-resistant and I have normal blood sugar levels, I can easily switch back and forth between sugar and fat burning. If you're diabetic, prediabetic, or have insulin resistance, you will probably want to stay in ketosis and not cycle in and out like I do. The ketogenic diet has been shown to cure type 2 diabetes, but that doesn't mean you can switch back to your old way of eating once you're cured.

THE COMMON DENOMINATOR

In chapter 8, Education, I'll introduce you to the DIG method that I learned from Dr. David Friedman, the author of *Food Sanity*. But I do want to bring out one point here before we get to that: your wellness choices should make sense to you. Just as things that seem too good to be true likely are, the things that seem stupid are probably wrong for you.

I've interviewed many authors on all sides of the diet spectrum—vegan, vegetarian, Mediterranean, low-FODMAP, Paleo, raw Paleo, ketogenic, and fasting. Because I'm a diet agnostic, I am able to learn from all of them. Over the years, I have found one common thread that ties them all together: they all agree that we are much better off if we eat high-quality, whole foods.

M&M'S ARE TECHNICALLY VEGETARIAN, BUT...

I knew someone who was a strict vegetarian, and she was morbidly obese. How could this be? I'll tell you.

She ate palmfuls of M&M's every day, a perfectly vegetarian-friendly food. Paleo, ketogenic, vegan—whatever form your nutrition plan takes, you should focus on getting the best quality, whole, unprocessed foods. Just because it fits your eating profile doesn't mean it's good for you. Choose well.

If your great-grandmother were to walk through a grocery store today, she would not recognize most of the items they sell. This is even true for Whole Foods, Trader Joe's, or any other "health food" store. In fact, it's really embarrassing that we have to use the term *whole food*. Whole food is really just food—real, unprocessed food.

So what is high-quality whole food? Here is a basic guide to help you determine whether your food choices are improving your wellness:

- Do you recognize it as a plant or animal? (Hint: bagels don't grow on trees.)
- If you left it out for over forty-eight hours, would it still look and taste good? (Hint: nature is not good at preserving things after they die or get picked.)
- Is it in a box, bag, or can? (Hint: real food doesn't have a nutrition label.)

- Does it have more frequent flyer miles than you do? (Hint: use Google Maps to see how far Ecuador is from your hometown and imagine how long it would take your produce to travel that distance by truck or boat.)
- Does the chicken breast look like it came from a chicken that could kick your butt? (Hint: chickens aren't bodybuilders and they don't need steroids. A normal chicken breast is about three to four ounces, not three-quarters of a pound.)
- Can your strawberry survive the zombie apocalypse? (Hint: bugs eat plants, too. Your produce should not be so toxic that bugs won't eat them.)
- Can you read through the ingredients list in one breath? (Hint: how many ingredients are there in organic kale? Or a grass-fed ribeye steak?)
- Does your produce look like it could win a Guinness World Record? (Hint: plants grow slow and deep to get nutrition from the soil. Short of this, they aren't as nutrient-rich. Fertilizers make them grow fast and big.)
- How was the animal raised? (Hint: chickens are not vegetarians. They love eating bugs. You can say, "Ew," but chickens on bug-based diets make the eggs much more nutritious and tasty.)

Yes, I had a little fun with that, but good nutrition is actually serious business. That said, I'm reminded of a conversation I had with Dr. Eric Westman, who runs HEAL Clinics, where he treats patients for diabetes and obesity. He recommends that everyone start down the road toward improving nutrition by reducing carbs and processed foods. Then, one step at a time, work to remove steroid- and antibiotic-laden meats, pesticide- and fertilizer-poisoned vegetables, preservatives and additives, and other chemicals that rob the nutrition from the food you eat.

A small step in the right direction is actually a huge step toward wellness.

For me, the quickest and simplest path to nutrition is to shop at the farmers market. I can learn about the food I'm eating, how and where it was raised or grown, and then I know I'm getting high-quality food. I can talk to the man or woman who runs the farm. Short of that, I'd recommend you do the vast majority of your shopping around the perimeter of the grocery store. That's where you'll find the vegetables, meat, fish, and eggs (just skip the bakery).

Eventually, you'll learn to see things that differentiate high-quality, whole food from the imposter foods. For example: an egg yolk should be orange, not yellow. When a chicken lives in the open and eats what chickens were intended to eat—such as seeds, bugs, and small critters—

they get better nutrition. Their own nutritional diet is reflected in a beautiful orange yolk.

HEALTH ENEMY NUMBER ONE: SUGAR AND REFINED CARBS

As you walk through a big grocery store, you see boxes, bags, and cans of carbohydrates everywhere you go. Even some canned meats have added sugars. If you look at the nutrition labels, you'll understand how the average American consumes 157 pounds of sugar every year. In the 1800s, that number was about two pounds per person per year.[10] And refined carbohydrates are just as bad.

Eating more sugar or refined carbs than you need at any given moment is like overfilling your gas tank, except instead of spilling the excess fuel on the pavement, your body triggers insulin to mop up the excess and stores it as body fat.

---

10   "Sugar and Sweeteners Yearbook Tables," United States Department of Agriculture, https://www.ers.usda.gov/data-products/sugar-and-sweeteners-yearbook-tables.aspx.

Your stomach is not your fuel tank—your muscles, liver, and blood are. When those body parts have all the fuel (sugar in the form of glycogen and blood glucose) you need, the rest has to be stored as fat. If you put eighty times more fuel into your car than the tank can carry, you'd have a real mess. Similarly, when you eat eighty times more sugar than you need, you have a metabolic disaster in your body. That's the effect of the standard American diet. How's that for SAD?

This is why we have an epidemic of type 2 diabetes, heart disease, Alzheimer's, and of course, obesity in America: overconsumption of sugar and processed foods.

As you start paying more attention to your gas gauge—and the type of and amount of gas you're putting in your car—you'll stop settling for cut-rate fuel. If your engine needs premium fuel, such as wild-caught fish and locally sourced organic vegetables, you'll make sure you go to the farmers market or the local co-op to get it. It might seem like it costs a lot more, but I assure you it is much cheaper than dialysis or a heart bypass surgery.

YOU EAT MORE SUGAR THAN YOU REALIZE

Every few months on my podcast, I like to run a twenty-eight-day sugar challenge, where we all cut our sugar intake. The beginner level is fifty grams a day. Everybody looks at that number, thinking keeping their intake below that will be no problem. Then they start actually logging their sugar intake—most sugar challenge participants realize they were consuming 200 to 300 grams a day. It is a challenge, but they quickly see how much better they look and feel when they get off the sugar.

Use a nutrition tracker such as MyFitnessPal to see how much sugar you're eating on a day-to-day basis. You might be surprised.

My clients quickly realize that my approach—while soft in tone—is firm in resolve. I hold them accountable, so when they go off their eating plan, I'm going to ask why.

The two reasons I get most are:

1. It costs too much money.
2. I didn't have time.

Both are BS excuses.

Yes, grocery stores will charge more for organic (it actually costs more to grow and raise), but when you eat more nutritious foods, you need less of them to get what you need. I'm going to let that sink in for a moment.

Because you get what you need nutritionally from whole foods, you're more satiated and you eat less.

Telling me you don't have time to eat well is like telling your spouse you didn't have time to buy them an anniversary gift. If you don't have time, you make time. And if not, I'm sure they'll understand—not!

You can dice up some chicken and stir-fry it in a healthy fat with bell peppers, spinach, and garlic in just twenty minutes. The crockpot is a must-have in my kitchen (we have four or five of them). I can put in a roast with tomatoes, bell peppers, and onions; add a half cup of red wine and some spices; and set it on low. Then we'll have a wonderful dinner ready six to eight hours later. And while I'm less familiar with the Instant Pot, I keep hearing it's also a great timesaver in the kitchen.

You can save even more time if you condense your cooking into a batch. I'm a huge fan of batch cooking. Spend one weekend afternoon making a large quantity of two or three healthy meals and parse it out in single-serving containers to eat throughout the week. Freeze what you won't eat just then, and pull it out the day before you need it.

You can even turn batch cooking into a bonding event with your friends and family. Invite them to join you. Let them know this is about eating healthy whole-food meals, so there will be no boxes, bags, or cans allowed. This can be a great way to discover new recipes while still spending quality time together.

Food should be enjoyed with others, and that includes the preparation.

THE DORITO EFFECT

Food companies have made a science around getting us addicted to junk food. Jeff Scot Philips, author of *Big Fat Food Fraud*, and Mark Schatzker, author of *The Dorito Effect*, were both guests on my podcast, and they discovered a terrifying secret of the food industry: companies are systematically forced to work through and around regulations to make food as tasty, sweet, and crunchy as can be. Their job is to literally make us crave more food.

Being good fiduciaries for the company's investors, they want you to eat more of their products, and they're very,

very good at their job. Because food companies can raise the prices only so much before people will switch to another brand, they have to keep us coming back for more. That's why you see twenty different Doritos flavors; a few dozen Pringles flavors; and cases of Bud Light Lime, Bud Light Orange, and I'm pretty sure a Bud Light Chocolate is in the works.

THREE CHIPS AT THE SAME TIME

Here is a perfect example: Pringles had a Super Bowl commercial where three guys each had a different flavor of chips: pizza, chicken, and barbecue. The protagonist (aka victim) ate his pizza chip and apparently loved it. His friend then gave him a chicken-flavored chip, which he stacked on a pizza chip. He ate the combo and said, "Mmm, chicken pizza." Then he got a chip from both friends, and stacked them. "Oh, barbecue chicken pizza!" They already make their chips taste really, really good, but the underlying message of this ad was to eat them three at a time.

Food is meant to give us the energy and nutrients to do the activities that bring us closer to wellness. Food is also the building block of our body. Imagine I let you choose between two cars: one made of high-grade metals and fiberglass, or one made with corkboard and plastic. Which one would you choose? Of course you'd pick the metal and fiberglass car—we want our cars to be made with high-quality materials for durability. The same holds true with your body.

So what do you think you're building your body with when you eat Pringles three at a time?

I'm sure you've heard the statement, "You are what you eat." It seems cliché, but it is 100 percent true. Over time, your body replaces all the cells in your body with new cells. The material used to make those new cells is coming from your food. If you haven't already, now is the time to start giving your body the best materials possible so you can be healthy and well.

MAKE YOUR OWN FOOD IRRESISTIBLE

Beyond making food taste great, natural herbs and spices give food even more health benefits. Turmeric, ginger, rosemary, and oregano have all been shown to be good for your health. Don't be fooled by the folks who tell you to eat a five-gallon bucket of the stuff to get an effective dose. Enjoy sprinkling these healthy spices on your food and enjoy the health benefits and the great taste!

Please don't let the food companies take your health hostage. Beyond making the food taste irresistible, they put a lot of thought into marketing. They use phrases such as "all-natural," "fortified," and "heart healthy" to convince you you're making a good, healthy choice. These are all marketing gimmicks. A ripe zucchini or a fresh apple doesn't have a label, but you know it's good for you. High-quality, healthy food doesn't need to market itself.

Love yourself enough to say no to fake food and yes to whole, unprocessed foods.

> ## BACON IS AMAZING! VERSUS BACON WILL KILL YOU!
>
> In stark contrast to my previous career as an internal auditor—where conflict was my bread and butter—I don't press the guests on my podcast as much as I could. I look for the nuggets of actionable tactics my listeners can benefit from and continue the interview. For me, it's more important to help my listeners than it is to challenge a guest to a debate in order to prove a point. That doesn't help anyone.
>
> As I write this, I'm reminded of some advice for married men that I learned many years ago. It goes like this: Would you rather be right or would you rather be happy? Because you can't be both. It makes me happy to bring value to my listeners, so I am not joining the "us versus them" food fight that is raging online through podcasts, blogs, and social media.
>
> 1. To vegans: How can we accept a way of eating that requires supplementation in order to be successful?
>
> 2. To the cholesterol alarmists: Isn't my body fat a saturated fat? Why is it OK to use my own body fat for energy but not to eat meat that has the same kind of fat?
>
> 3. To ketogenic people: Can we stop pushing bacon as a primary food for the ketogenic diet? It's processed, packaged, and should not be considered a core component of our diet.

Beyond providing fuel and building materials, the third purpose of food is to be enjoyable. Eating food should be a pleasurable event, a celebration even. Thanksgiving, Christmas, Easter, the end of Ramadan—they're all food-centered celebrations. It's an awesome experience when we derive joy from food without it forcing us down the detours to poor health.

Use food to spend time with your friends and family, whether it's batch cooking, going to the farmers market, or sitting down to eat a healthy meal together.

Food is your energy source, the building blocks of your body, and a source of joy. As you go down the road to wellness, you'll want to keep putting better and better fuel in your engine and upgrading the components you use to build your vehicle. You'll also want to bring along some passengers and sing along to the radio. Food should be one of the best parts of your wellness journey.

HYDRATION

Most of us spend much of our lives in some form of dehydration simply because we don't make drinking water a priority. Likewise, coffee, alcohol, and many prescription drugs act as diuretics, which dehydrate us more. It's time to set your sights on POW: plain old water.

Water serves many purposes in the body. Do you remember those old biochemical batteries in cars? You had to add water to them to keep them functioning well. You definitely need to add water to your body for the same reason.

Good hydration helps keep your joints well lubricated so you can move without wearing them out. Just as dry and cracked belts and hoses are an issue for your car, dry cartilage in your knees and back can leave you broken down and stranded.

If you're working to lose weight (in the form of body fat), make sure you drink plenty of water. When your liver gets hit with too many toxins, it will take many of those toxins and store them in your fat cells. It's sneaky but effective. However, now that you're burning that fat, the toxins come out and it's the kidneys' job to deal with them. Your kidneys need water to flush those toxins out of your body. Give your kidneys the water they need to do this very important job.

HOW MANY GLASSES OF WATER A DAY?

You've likely heard that you need eight glasses of water per day, but did you know there is no science to back that claim? So how much water do you actually need each day? Well, it depends.

Much of it will depend on your environment. Both hot weather and very cold weather cause us to lose hydration.

Likewise, when you sweat through a tough workout, you need to replace the water you lose through the sweat. And you've probably noticed how your skin gets dry during very cold weather. This is another circumstance in which you need to increase your water intake.

Vegetables and fruits can provide you with a lot of hydration. However, if you're eating ketogenic—where you're eating fewer carbs—I'd encourage you to increase your water intake.

If you find yourself feeling hungry between meals, it might mean you need more water. We often misinterpret the thirst signal as hunger. Before you eat a snack, try drinking a big glass of water and see if the hunger goes away.

THE TRUE TEST OF HYDRATION

How can you tell if you're properly hydrated? You can gauge your hydration level by checking out your urine: it should be mostly clear with only a hint of yellow. If your urine is deep yellow or brownish, you're dehydrated. This test doesn't work if you're taking a B-vitamin complex, which may make your pee look like a lightsaber. In that case, you'll want to use my second test.

Check out your skin. Your skin looks and feels better if you properly hydrate. Take some time each morning to check your skin. If it's dry and flaky, your insides might be a bit dry, too. Help them out with a big glass of water.

WHERE TO GET YOUR WATER

My county government pumps potable water into my house, I turn on the faucet, and it comes out. Perfect, right? Well, some studies show that the fluoride in tap water can be a health risk. They add fluoride to prevent tooth decay, but because you're not eating sugar, guess what? Tooth decay isn't a big risk for you. A good filter can remove the fluoride if you're concerned about it.

And yes, some tests have even found chemicals and medications in municipal water supplies. It is a growing problem, and I'm hopeful they figure out how to make tap water safer, but that shouldn't stop you from getting the water you need.

I remember the first time I bought a bottle of water at a convenience store. I looked at the price in shock: it cost the same as a soft drink? *How?* I reluctantly paid the price anyway because I needed water.

In most stores these days, you'll see multiple brands available for purchase. What most people don't realize is that despite the name on the label, most of the water brands are just repackaged (and maybe filtered) tap water.

Beyond the price and the fact that it's just repackaged tap water, there are two core issues with bottled water. For a start, most of the bottles are made with a chemical called bisphenol-a (BPA), which can seep into the water. This chemical disrupts our sex hormones, particularly estrogen, which is not good for either men or women. The second issue is that plastic bottles are single-use items. Most of them end up in landfills or, worse, as pollution in our lakes, rivers, and oceans.

So a good hydration strategy would entail buying a stainless steel water bottle, and either using bulk spring water (they come in one-gallon and five-gallon jugs) or water filtered with a high-quality filter to refill it. This solution will address most of the issues I mentioned above.

Water is life. Start drinking the water you need today, even if it's out of your tap or from a bottle. You can always work on improving the quality of your water as you go.

And before you ask: no, soft drinks DO NOT count toward your hydration.

Soft drinks are ubiquitous in the United States. They're in convenience stores, restaurants, vending machines, and in rows and rows in grocery stores. I used to be addicted to Diet Coke (yes, soft drinks are addictive). All of them— Coke, Pepsi, Mountain Dew, Sprite, and Dr. Pepper—are nothing more than sugar bombs. When you drink soda, you may as well tell your liver and pancreas to fire up the fat-making process, because that's where most of your soda is likely to go.

Maybe you think the diet versions are better. Let me stop you right there. I've never heard of *anyone* who lost weight because they switched from regular soda to the zero-calorie version. In fact, most of us just get fatter drinking diet soda because we think it's good for us and drink more. Plus the diet drinks are sweetened with chemicals such as aspartame, saccharin, and sucralose. When we introduce our body to a chemical it doesn't recognize, we can usually expect it to do something very bad for our health.

THE TRUTH ABOUT STEVIA

When my wife, Tammy, and I were first dating, she was at my apartment and she went into the spice cabinet for salt. Inside of the cabinet, she found a baggie with dried green leaves. She turned to me holding the bag and said, "What the hell is this?" What she thought was an illegal substance was actually stevia.

On a trip to Argentina, I was introduced to stevia and yerba mate tea. When used in yerba mate, stevia makes an excellent sweetener—I could let them steep together and the result would be a very mellow, sweet tealike drink. Unfortunately, my yerba mate had recently run out, and I was not able to find another good use for the natural stevia. It is very sweet, but it has a bitter tinge to it. That's why it was sitting forgotten in my spice cupboard.

Soon after that moment with Tammy in my apartment, I started noticing stevia in grocery stores everywhere. But what I saw was not the stevia I knew. To make it useful as a sweetener, companies process it into a white powder. They add ingredients to offset the bitterness, and they add fillers to bulk it up and make it comparable in volume to the competing artificial sweeteners. Essentially, what they've done is taken a natural product and created a Frankenfood.

If you can, it's best to avoid all of the drinks that have sugar, artificial sweeteners, and even natural sweeteners. Just stick to POW.

Drinking water is not enough, however. In order for your body to *utilize* water, you need to give yourself the proper electrolytes, such as sodium and potassium. Without consuming enough electrolytes, even drinking gallons of water won't keep you hydrated. I wish I had known that during a trip to Malaysia.

SOUTHEAST ASIA

Over the course of the many years when I was trying to figure out my wellness roadmap, I went through cycles when I'd get a spurt of inspiration and I'd go gung-ho about my health and fitness. During one of those gung-ho spurts, I went on a business trip to Malaysia. Malaysia is a beautiful country, but it is very hot and humid, even early in the mornings. Despite the weather, I got up every morning and sweated my butt off running outside. Sweat is just fat crying as it leaves your body, right?

It happened to be Ramadan during my visit, which is their fasting month. They didn't eat from sunrise to sunset for an entire month. Out of respect for my coworkers and staff, I opted to participate, at least partially. I'd eat my breakfast, skip lunch, and then eat a small dinner. I was drinking lots of water—to keep myself feeling full throughout the day.

I don't like to eat on airplanes—it always makes me feel bloated—so on the twenty-six hours of flights home, I didn't eat. I just pounded down bottle after bottle of water.

It was a perfect "diet" week, during which I lost ten

pounds. I felt like I'd done something wonderful for my health with this "move more, eat less" approach.

I was wrong.

I was fine throughout the trip, during the flight, and even the first two nights after getting home.

Then, three days later, it hit me. I was sitting at my desk at work and all of a sudden I got the shakes. The shakes turned to convulsions, and the pain in my stomach sent me to the floor. I threw up and defecated as I shook on the ground. I was an absolute mess and I had no idea what was happening. Despite my coworkers wanting to call an ambulance, I decided not to go to the hospital. I just cleaned my office and myself the best I could and went home.

By nine o'clock that evening, I finally checked my ego. My chest hurt, and I had an eerie feeling that something was seriously wrong. I drove myself to the hospital.

When you tell an ER nurse that you have chest pains, they don't mess around. They gave me nitroglycerin, put me on an IV, and took some blood samples. An hour or so later, a nurse came back and gave me the results.

"It is not a heart attack. You're extremely dehydrated," he

said. "But that's not the only problem. Your electrolytes are low—off-the-charts low. Your sodium is bad enough that you could have gone into a coma."

By not having enough potassium and sodium in my diet, I wasn't able to hold on to the water in my body, even though I was drinking a ton of it. Sodium helps keep water in your body, and potassium helps keep water in your cells. Both are critical for good hydration. Because I was drinking so much water, I washed those electrolytes out of my system, dropping my levels even lower. I got what is known as hyponatremia, or water poisoning.

We all like simple rules, such as "Drink eight glasses of water per day," but you have to make sure your body has a way to use that water, meaning you need to get adequate electrolytes such as sodium and potassium (I'll throw magnesium in there as well because it is an electrolyte, and it is involved in so many functions in the body).

That was a brutal learning experience, but I educated myself to understand how my body works: my sodium and potassium levels run low. Now, using that experience as a learning moment, I diligently track my electrolytes with my quarterly blood work. I also eat foods that have the nutrients I need, such as sodium, potassium, and magnesium, and I use Himalayan sea salt to make sure I'm getting what my body needs.

While we don't start out with a user manual, you can use life events like I did and others' experiences to better understand yourself. That's when you'll start crafting your own user manual, and you'll improve your wellness due to the educational experiences life gives you and your willingness to act on what you learn.

CHAPTER 8

EDUCATION

Only a year ago, I still had my incredibly stressful job as the head of internal audit for a major corporation. We were going through a third year of significant downsizing. Being a manager in that environment was extremely stressful because, yes, while my own position was in jeopardy, I was very concerned about the well-being of the other hardworking people in my department.

Our department dwindled over those three years, from twenty-three to fifteen, to twelve, nine, and eventually zero—all of us were laid off. It was gut-wrenchingly hard and stressful to have those "You're done" conversations. I hope I never have to hear about "head counts" as they relate to people's livelihood ever again.

This happened over my fall feasting season, so while it was normal for me to put on a little bit of weight that time of year, I had never packed on pounds like I did that fall. Like I said before, I normally add about ten to fifteen pounds over the fall, but that year I put on twenty-five pounds—all due to the stress.

I knew I needed to get a grasp on my stress. Fortunately, through the 40+ *Fitness Podcast*, I have access to the best experts in every health-related field I can imagine. I reached out to several stress experts, read their books, and then interviewed them for the podcast.

A lot of people would have said it was the food that was causing me to gain weight, and they wouldn't have been entirely wrong. Stress trumped everything else I did for my wellness. Through my conversations with stress experts and by learning the quirks of my vehicle, I knew that the real problem was stress. The side effects of the stress just happened to manifest as poor choices and weight gain.

I found myself dealing with the stress of layoffs by using alcohol and bad food, neither of which was the right answer. I had to find a healthy, more sustainable coping mechanism to deal with the fact that I still had to tell eight other people, some of whom I'd worked with for more than a decade, that they no longer had jobs. Oh, did I mention this was during December? Merry Christmas.

Through my wellness education, I learned a method called

3-4-5 breathing from Dr. Rangan Chatterjee, author of *How to Make Disease Disappear*. In short, the 3-4-5 method means you breathe in for three seconds, hold for four seconds, and breathe out for five seconds. (I'd originally learned this as box breathing, but I like Dr. Chatterjee's version better.) This breathing method has been a huge piece of ammunition in my stress relief arsenal.

Mindfully counting your breath in and out helps you be fully present in the moment—it forces you to focus on your breathing, and in that way, it helps clear your mind. When I first tried it, it worked. In stressful moments, I could utilize this breathing technique to recenter myself and handle the intensity of that time in my life.

As an example, whenever my boss called me up to his office, I felt a surge of cortisol that sent me into a full fight-or-flight response. I didn't have the time to do my regular stress management activity (going to the gym and throwing around heavy weights), so using the 3-4-5 breathing method was just what I needed.

I needed to teach myself a method to deal with stress that I could do in the elevator on my way up to my boss's office. I could have the meeting without feeling like I needed to smash something or sprint away. Then, after the meeting, I could finally head over to the gym and rid myself of the remaining cortisol in my system.

This new practice I learned through my wellness education gave me a powerful tool to better manage my stress. (We will talk more about stress in chapter 10, Stress Management.)

Do you remember the big rocks, little rocks, and sand exercise I told you about in chapter 4? Early on, you may find that you have a lot of big rocks sitting in front of you. That's a daunting image, but it's actually a good situation to be in—it means you have a lot of opportunity in front of you to improve your wellness. I'd like to give you a little guidance on finding your biggest rocks first and educating yourself to successfully place them in your jar.

GAUGES ON THE DASHBOARD

If you look at the dash of your car, you'll see a few gauges that require your attention. Each gauge gives you information about your vehicle's ability to get you to your destination. We can relate these gauges to four key elements of wellness: training, rest, food, and stress.

Let's go through the gauges on your dash and how you can relate them to your body and your wellness journey.

GAS GAUGE

I remember driving my Jeep from Houston to Austin with

my daughter. As I drove down the highway, I forgot to pay attention to the gas gauge. When I finally looked down, it was on empty, and I wasn't sure I'd make it to the next gas station. Luckily, we made it to an exit, but right as I pulled into the station, the engine died. Fortunately, I was able to coast up to the pump.

Nobody wants to run out of gas, particularly on the highway. Food is your fuel, and it's the most important gauge on your car's dashboard. By monitoring your energy level and how certain foods affect you, you can get an idea of how well you're fueling your wellness.

OIL GAUGE

I made a point of keeping my Jeep healthy by getting regular oil changes. One time when I got my oil changed, I noted my oil light was still on as I pulled out of the shop. I immediately turned the ignition off and checked the oil. They forgot to do the most important part of an oil change: they didn't replace the oil in my car!

Your oil level is easy to overlook, as is sleep and rest. If you neglect your oil, you'll destroy your car. Fatigue and sleep deprivation will likewise keep you from reaching your wellness vision.

HEAT GAUGE

My Jeep had a tendency of running hot—it was a quirk of the model. I had to be doubly aware of my engine temperature when it was a hot day or I was driving down steep mountain roads. I had to change my driving style and occasionally pull over and let the car cool down.

Your heat gauge measures your stress level. (We will cover stress more in depth in chapter 10, Stress Management.) When you train, you are stressing your body in order to coax it to grow. If work or family issues also stress you, you risk overheating. You may need to let up on your training intensity or pull over and cool down.

VOLTAGE GAUGE

My Jeep never had issues keeping a charge, so my voltage meter was always in range. Unfortunately, I can't say the same for my training. I have had times when I trained way too hard and times when I didn't train enough.

If you don't run your car regularly, your battery loses its charge—training actually gives us the necessary voltage to continue down the highway to fitness. Too much training and your voltage skyrockets, causing you to blow out your battery. Just as a car's alternator is set to charge the twelve-volt battery at fourteen volts, you should train at a point just beyond your comfort zone.

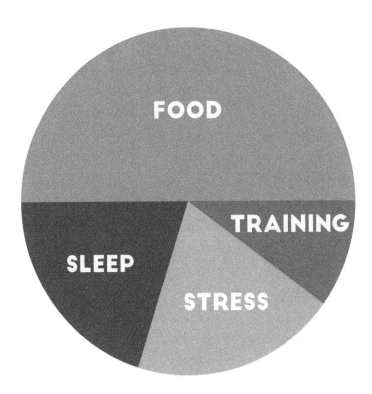

CAN YOU DIG IT?

I recently interviewed the author of *Food Sanity*, Dr. David Friedman. In his book, Dr. Friedman introduced a very useful technique to weed out bad science about foods. It's called the DIG method, which stands for Discovery, Instinct, and God. While he developed DIG to address the science of food, I think it is a great tool to educate yourself about any tactic you want to use on your wellness journey.

DISCOVERY

In my mid-twenties, I could barely wait for each issue of *Muscle and Fitness* to come out. That magazine was full of tactics and nutrition plans that the pros were supposedly using. I remember one plan called 100s, where you do one hundred reps of an exercise, such as barbell curls. There were no science references in the article, just an endorsement from a famous-at-the-time bodybuilder saying it worked for him. In my opinion, the 100s exercise plan was potentially dangerous—it was an easy way to completely fry your muscles—and it had zero science to back it up.

As you educate yourself about your wellness, you should continue to tread cautiously. Even if you find educational materials with scientific sources, don't be fooled by the MD after the source's name. Doctors want to make money, too.

I recently listened to a podcast where a doctor described a supplement called glutathione that would make the liver super-resilient. Glutathione can be a valuable supplement. However, he then began boasting that you wouldn't get superdrunk or have hangovers when taking it. He was even helpful enough to discuss the best type of glutathione to take. Sounds great, huh?

It just so happens that he was describing a supplement

that he sells. He had a concrete motivation for pushing his own supplement, and it's less likely he wanted what was best for your wellness.

If, however, in the discovery process you find that a tactic is actually based on something more solid than someone's uninformed opinion or a sales pitch, then you can move on to the next filter.

INSTINCT

Use your common sense as you educate yourself. Does the information you're reading or hearing *make sense?*

I recently followed some discussions on a health-focused Facebook group where a man was experimenting with dry fasts, meaning he went twenty-four hours or more without drinking water. He saw a fitness "guru" on YouTube touting the miracle benefits of a dry fast, so off he went. That was an incredibly dangerous and reckless wellness choice he made—all because he didn't use his common sense.

GOD

Finally, ask yourself if your chosen tactic aligns with your belief in yourself and your relationship with the universe, whatever form that might take. A study might come out saying pork is the best meat you can eat, but if you're Jewish or Muslim, then it doesn't matter how good pork is for you—it still won't align with your belief system. For a tactic to work, you have to apply it consistently over a long time. That won't be easy if it doesn't jibe with who you are.

Dr. Friedman's DIG method is a great system to analyze if a new tactic you discover through your education is truly worth considering. If you find a tactic that actually addresses one of your bigger rocks and it passes the DIG evaluation, then you're on to experimentation.

EXPERIMENTATION

I interviewed at least six different authors to educate myself on stress management, and they all gave me different tactics and approaches to address my problem. I had to experiment to find what worked best for me. Even for someone with a ton of experience, the overabundance of health advice out there can be overwhelming and confusing.

Go to Google and enter "weight loss without workout" and you'll get more than four million results. It's an absolute muck. After people wrote the first ten, why did anyone bother writing the next 3,999,990? They're just giving you even more tactics.

I specifically avoided making this a book about tactics, because I know that a good wellness *mindset* is the only thing that will keep you on path. Strategies will help you avoid the pitfalls and challenges, and then you can look for the tactics to help you overcome them. But you must proceed in that order: mindset, then strategies, and then tactics.

STRATEGIES VERSUS TACTICS

It's easy to confuse strategies and tactics. I like to think of them like this: strategies are the things we do to make sure we reach our wellness vision, whereas tactics are the things we do to get and stay well.

For example, as a strategy, I prepare my workout clothes and leave my gym bag by the door the night before. The tactics I use include any supplements I take (e.g., creatine) and the type of workout I do in the gym. My strategy ensures I get to the gym consistently, and the tactics get me the results I want.

Once you have your path charted and you're on your way down your wellness path, then yes, tactics matter. That's why I work hard to get some actionable advice from each expert I interview on the *40+ Fitness Podcast*. But always remember: tactics are just tools in your wellness toolbox.

In order to fix your car, you have to not only choose the

right tool, but you also have to know how to use it. That's what experimentation helps you discover: which tactics work *for you* and how to use them.

Most of the articles and books you read about wellness will tell you only the equivalent of how to use your turn signal. I'm telling you to figure out which direction you want to turn. Your car's GPS may say, "In half a mile, turn left," or if you have the Waze app, it's Mr. T yelling, "Turn left, fool." When you know you need to turn left, by all means use that turn signal (the tactic) to ensure you can do so safely. Just know that not all tactics work like a good turn signal—some of them will be a waste of time for you.

Spaghetti against the Wall

After I've been doing the same workout for eight weeks, I'll typically see my strength plateau. That's when I know I need to change something up. I can use that time to learn different training programs, like the ones I'd find in Dr. Doug McGuff's book, *Body by Science*, or Mark Rippetoe's book, *Starting Strength*. I could try out one of their training programs and see how it works for me.

But I won't just walk into a new training regimen blindly. A good experiment has a hypothesis. You're not using the "spaghetti against the wall" method, where you just keep throwing things out there to see what sticks. You have to be *intentional* with your changes. Experimenting just for the sake of it won't do you any good.

First ask yourself if this tactic addresses a big rock. Then run it through the DIG test. If it still holds up, it's just a matter of trying it out and giving it enough time for you to see a result.

For example, I worked with one client who wanted stronger legs. He'd been improving his squats considerably, but he was beginning to plateau because of confidence issues as he increased the amount of weight on the bar. He knew he could get down into the squat; he just didn't know if he'd be able to get up.

I told him we needed to switch lanes and do a seated leg press on a machine for six weeks. It's a controlled move, where he'd have much more control over the weight and wouldn't feel as exposed. Through that experiment, he was able to continue improving his strength, which helped boost his confidence.

Lo and behold, when he came back to the squat rack, he started lifting much more weight—he'd busted through the plateau. He learned a new tactic (with the help of his trainer) and experimented with it. It was a successful experiment that got him back into the fast lane on his wellness journey.

The human body is a wonderful and complex machine. We can improve it when we eat the right foods, get good quality rest and sleep, manage our stress, and train it with proper progression. But there is no one-size-fits-all solution for anything wellness related. You have to experiment to find what works best for *you*. That's what we call an n = 1 experiment.

FAILED EXPERIMENTS

I explained earlier in the book that when you experiment with your health and wellness, you're doing an experiment where you are the only subject. An n = 1 experiment is a process by which you try a tactic, give it time to show its results, and analyze what you discover. Most of your n = 1 experiments will reward you with better health and fitness, but some of them will fail.

MY N = 1 FAILURE: THE STATIN STORY

Before I ever tried to fix my cholesterol with the pescatarian diet, I experimented with my doctor's recommendation to take statins. The resulting side effects were so bad I knew I'd never go back. Here's what happened.

A friend and I decided to train for the Bataan Death March race, a tribute to prisoners of war in the Philippines who marched without food or water for seventy-six miles, many of whom died on the march. It's basically a marathon through the New Mexico desert. Sound appealing? It gets better: the participants are actually *encouraged* to wear a thirty-five-pound backpack as a sign of respect for the weight the American soldiers carried.

Around the same time I started training for the race, my doctor put me on statins for my cholesterol. (Remember how I told you to always check with your doctor before starting a new training program? Yes, I actually follow my own advice.)

I had no idea how badly I'd respond to the statins.

One day, I loaded my backpack with fifteen pounds of books and went for a walk with my daughter, Bekah, who was seven at the time. We were about a half mile from our house when all of a sudden my legs locked up. All of my muscles seized, and I went to the ground.

"Daddy," Bekah said, "are you OK?"

I couldn't stand up.

This was supposed to be the practice of my vision: I was spending time doing something active with my daughter. I wanted her to see me as a healthy and fit father. Instead, I was lying on the side of the road a half mile from the house, in severe pain, with no idea how we would possibly get back.

After several minutes, I was able to get on my feet and slowly walk home with Bekah. I got into my truck and went back for the backpack, defeated.

The statins had robbed me of my ability to train. I couldn't do the walks with a backpack, let alone any running or weight lifting. When I called the doctor about this little incident, he called in a prescription for a different statin. It was just more of the same for me—I still couldn't train. A week later, I called my doctor again and told him I would never take a statin ever again.

My friend and I never did make it out to New Mexico for the Bataan Death March. That still bothers me to this day.

That was my experience with statins: my muscles shut down, and I was actively deprived of my wellness vision.

(If you read the warning label on most statins, muscle locking is a common side effect for many people.)

I tried statins with an open mind and I did my n = 1 experiment. It failed. While the actual results of the experiment were not good, I learned an important lesson: statins didn't bring me closer to my vision—they took me further away from it.

Don't be discouraged by failed experiments; they can be just as valuable as the ones that work.

ARE YOU AN ELITE ATHLETE?

Some elite athletes wear masks that emulate lower oxygen levels, simulating high-altitude air. It helps them achieve perhaps a single percent improvement on their endurance. Now, for an elite athlete, that small performance gain can mean the difference between last place and first place. But for the rest of us, these little rocks and sand can be a huge distraction. Over the years, I've spent (OK, wasted) thousands of dollars on gadgets, tools, and apps that amounted to nothing more than sand. Even worse, I wasted time on experiments that weren't helping me get down the wellness road any faster.

Apply the tools in this chapter to have a better understanding of which tactics to try. Once you've worked through the big rocks and the little rocks, then you can experiment with sand like an altitude mask.

INJURIES AND FREAK STORMS

When I worked as an internal auditor, I would often employ the help of ethical hackers. What is an ethical hacker? Put simply, they're the same as the hackers you hear about on the news, but these folks help you *improve* the security of your systems by attempting to hack you and then telling you where your weaknesses are. As a result of their help, you can then fix your weaknesses, thus hardening your system.

But there's a new type of hacking that is sweeping across the internet, on podcasts, and in bookstores: the biohack.

The mere existence of biohacking as a wellness solution assumes that there are shortcuts on the wellness journey. That's science fiction.

The distance between Pensacola Beach and Philadelphia is fixed—there aren't any shortcuts. There might be an optimal route, which my GPS is likely to calculate as I go, but I still have to slog through what will be, at minimum, a seventeen-hour drive. I say "at minimum" because there are obstacles that could pop up to slow my journey.

Although we'd all like the road to wellness to be clear of obstacles, you'll inevitably run into problems. You'll need to stop to perform routine maintenance, fill up with gas, and perhaps you'll even run into rough weather.

An injury is like the freak thunderstorms we get down here in Florida. The rain pours down so hard you can't see the road, and you have to pull over. Even the folks who take the chance to keep driving only do so with their hazard lights on and traveling about thirty miles per hour on the freeway. This is similar to what happens when you get injured.

One of my freak storms came in the form of a torn rotator cuff. Years of wear and tear came to bite me one day when I was lifting weights. I had to pull off the road and get surgery, do rehab, and educate myself with new exercises so I could continue on the path to wellness.

Whatever is causing you to pull over to the side of the road—whether it's a torn rotator cuff or a cold that's keeping you from going to the gym—you have to accept it and move on. Now, that obstacle becomes your biggest rock. Pull over, deal with it, and once you know the storm is gone, safely get back on the highway and continue pushing onward.

SHAKING THE JAR

There's one important detail from the rocks-in-the-jar lesson that I want to cover before we finish this chapter: you have to shake the jar. Every time you put big rocks, little rocks, or sand in the jar—in other words, whenever you educate yourself enough to try a new tactic on your wellness journey—you have to shake the jar to let it settle. Another word for that is *action*. You must act on your education, and you must be consistent with your actions in order to run a proper n = 1 experiment.

The settling takes a little time. If you don't give your experiment enough time, you won't know whether it was truly successful or not. With some experiments, like the one I did with statins, the answer will come within days. Others may take weeks or months.

In the next chapter, we'll discuss this important concept—time—and everything you need to do to move down the road to wellness as efficiently as possible.

CHAPTER 9

TIME

I once had a troubling email correspondence with a podcast listener. She said, "I love your podcast. I've learned so much, and I'd like to learn more about training with you." Of course, I responded to her email, like I do with all of the *40+ Fitness Podcast* listeners, and I asked her the same thing I ask everyone who wants to work with me:

What are your health and fitness goals? What do you want to accomplish by working with me?

Her answer? "I need to lose seventy pounds for my daughter's wedding, which is in two months."

Now, don't get me wrong: anyone who has seventy pounds to lose can lose seventy pounds. It won't be easy, but it can be done, even in two months. There are plenty of trainers who would say, "Come on board; let's lose that weight," and they might even be successful, but I couldn't in good conscience take her as a client.

People see *The Biggest Loser* and think it's a realistic possibility to lose one hundred pounds in three months because someone on TV did it. Here's the part that most viewers overlook on the show. The trainers and producers do something very important that you can't replicate in the real world: they lock the contestants in a house with a limited amount of food. Then they work the contestants like mad. And they're under constant medical attention.

They're prisoners, in other words. They're voluntary prisoners, but prisoners nevertheless.

FAT IS AN ORGAN

My time in the Army as an infantry soldier was very similar to what the contestants on *The Biggest Loser* experience. Each bout of field training had me out in the woods or jungle for up to two weeks. I couldn't help but lose weight, even when I didn't have that much to lose. Three letters can explain my weight loss: M, R, and E. Those letters stand for "meal ready to eat," which is a meal in a packet that is standard issue in the US Army. Back in the eighties when I was active, each MRE contained a 1,000-calorie meal.

As a twenty-one-year-old out in the field, I was issued

three MREs a day, which equates to 3,000 calories. For most people, this would have been fine, but because I moved around so much, my body burned 6,500 or more calories a day. I can't begin to describe how that hunger felt.

Without access to any additional food, I had to improvise. Because I didn't drink coffee, I traded my coffee for other soldiers' creamer, cocoa, and sugar. I put the sugar in a creamer packet, mixed it up, and held it over a lighter. After about a minute, I had a little sugar cookie. I could also make some chocolate pudding with the cocoa powder. I made sure no food went to waste.

Still, I lost a pound for every day we were out there—not because I wanted to, but because I had no choice. I had limited access to food and I was required to move constantly. (So, yes, there is truth to the "calories in, calories out" model for weight loss. It's not the whole story, but calories do matter.)

When I came back from the field, my body didn't stay at this thinner, nearly emaciated form. It went back to normal, the same way the Biggest Losers' bodies return to their previous size.

Our bodies are designed to seek balance—equilibrium— so most *fast and extreme* changes to our bodies don't stick.

The reason is something called homeostasis. Homeostasis is a mechanism in your body through which it finds balance. While I pushed through the field training, my body adjusted to my new food reality, I needed to move, and food was scarce. When I got home and went back to eating like I had been before, my body used the opportunity to quickly return me to my previous "normal" weight.

Had we stayed out in the field for longer, my body would have adjusted. My weight would have stabilized and found a balance—homeostasis. With my return to my old eating style, I gave my body a clear signal that the famine was over and it was time to store fat.

Quick weight loss is not sustainable. It wasn't sustainable for me as an Army soldier in the field, it's not sustainable for *The Biggest Loser* contestants, and it's not sustainable for you either. That's why so many of those contestants gain it all back, and more, after the show.

That listener who emailed me didn't gain her weight in two months—she shouldn't have expected to *lose it* in two months and keep it off. That weight was a part of her. Fat isn't just a backpack or a spare tire you wear; it's an organ. It can shrink smaller as your body draws on the fat stores, but shrinking it too quickly will send a signal to your body that something is wrong. You have to find a gentle path and a safe pace if you want *sustainable* weight loss.

Gentle and safe is also what you'll want for every other facet of your vision. The road to wellness takes time.

THE THREE PS

When I work with clients with a big vision, one that I know they've bought into and believe in, I teach them about the three Ps to wellness: patience, persistence, and progression.

PATIENCE

Trying to bypass hard work and get straight to the results is like that kid in the back seat of a road trip asking, "Are we there yet? Are we there yet?" You've set your Wellness GPS. Even if your journey takes years, you will need patience and trust in the process.

F*%$!*$ SCALE

You already know I'm not a big fan of the scale, but I do understand the appeal of losing weight. So if you're set on reaching a given weight rather than a certain dress or pant size, one pound per week is a reasonable pace *if you have the body fat to spare.* But beware.

You might knock off four pounds the first week and two pounds the next week, but then you might *gain* half a pound the week after that. Don't get discouraged. The "one pound per week" isn't a linear progression, it's just an average. Look at your trend over time rather than your short-term fluctuations.

No matter what your wellness goal is, much of your journey is a process of undoing some bad habits from your past. In most cases, we've had those bad habits for decades and the results have accumulated over that time. Suppose you're driving and you take a wrong turn (I've done this so many times). Twenty minutes later, you discover your mistake. You turn the car around (making a legal U-turn, of course) and head back. It would be unreasonable to think you can get back to the point you lost your way in just a few minutes. It might not be a full twenty, but it will take time.

It will take time and patience for you to undo those bad habits and see real results. If you set your Wellness GPS, you will find your way and you'll make fewer wrong turns in the future. You can't live without the GPS when you're driving a new route.

In Lewis Carroll's *Alice's Adventures in Wonderland*, Alice talks to the Cheshire Cat. The cat says, "If you don't know where you're going, any road will get you there." You were likely on this health and fitness road for a while before you found this book. At the very least, you were thinking about it. Up until now, however, you haven't really known where you were going.

How well has wandering worked so far?

That's why we set our vision: to see where we're going. Your vision might be the next county over, or across the country, or in another country entirely. See the journey for what it is.

Some people travel the speed limit on the road to wellness, some people go really slowly, and others go so fast it seems like you're standing still. Trying to lose seventy pounds in two months is the equivalent of going thirty miles per hour over the speed limit. That technique might get you to your destination faster, but you're taking a lot of risks in the process. You could crash, you could get pulled over for speeding (injured), or you might just blow up your engine.

Take an honest assessment of the vehicle you're driving before you zoom off impatiently. When I was an Army recruit in my early twenties, I had a body that was like a sports car that was built to go fast over long periods. And even I injured myself.

You're most likely driving a slower car, one with much less horsepower than a younger, newer model. You have to ease into your fitness plan. You have to have patience. You won't do yourself any favors by accelerating up to eighty-five miles per hour, then overheating. Instead, look at the grand scheme—your vision—and ask if you're moving at a sustainable speed.

Find the balance between acceleration and a comfortable speed. You need to make wellness a sustainable lifestyle. Too often, people think of their wellness goals in terms of diets. A diet is a finite term—you go *on* a diet and then you go off it. I've seen many diet successes. Weight is lost, then what? They regain all of that weight and more.

You're not embarking on this journey toward wellness so you can come back. I don't think you planned this as a round trip. You have to set up your lifestyle so you never return to your origin.

If you check your weight regularly, then I'm sure you've experienced gaining a pound or two overnight. You were probably shocked and upset. In essence, the scale was calling you a diet failure. In those moments, you have to turn away from your emotions and turn on the logic. You didn't eat thousands of calories more than your body needed (3,500 calories = one pound of fat).

You most likely retained some water weight, not fat. Will that change in the number on the scale be the gust of wind that knocks your car off the road? Or will you have the patience to recognize it as an anomaly that has less to do with your actual progress and more to do with a random biological circumstance? Wellness takes time and patience. No matter where your journey takes you, your road to success will not be a straightaway. It's not a drag race.

PERSISTENCE

Imagine you're at the beginning of your wellness journey and you decide to eat keto. Monday through Thursday of this week, you did awesome: you ate exactly what was on your meal plan, you've been diligent about quantities and quality of food, and you can already feel yourself getting healthier. You're starting to show ketones on the urine stick.

Then Friday comes around and a coworker invites you out for happy-hour drinks. They choose a place that carries your favorite wine. "Screw it," you think, "I've been good all week. I'll just have two glasses and stop at that." You're sure you read somewhere that you can have wine with keto as long as you don't overdo it.

Then on Saturday, you go to a football tailgate and you have a bowl of chili. You applaud yourself for keeping away from all the other bad foods. You feel you've made the best choice. Then on Sunday, you're right back to your meal plans, batch cooking for the upcoming week with healthy meals. You feel good about the previous week, even though you cheated a few times—*the nice outweighed the naughty.*

You check your ketones on Sunday night—there is not a ketone to be found. What gives?

Although you started off great, you didn't maintain persistence over the course of the week. You were relying on willpower, rather than having built a healthy lifestyle. So when normal challenges popped up, such as the drinks after work or the tailgate on the weekend, you weren't ready to handle them.

There will be all kinds of distractions on the road to wellness. You'll see signs that say, "White alligator farm!" or "World's largest wooden beaver!" These signs draw your attention, tickle your imagination, and try to get you to take a detour.

A few distractions here and there can actually be good for you. For example, maybe you've been waiting your whole life to see the world's largest wooden beaver, so the benefit you'd derive from pulling off the road and taking a quick detour would be worth it for you, and you know you can get back on the road to wellness.

What if your spouse surprises you with a vacation to Hawaii after weeks of eating keto? This is your dream vacation! Are you going to say no? Are you going to visit Hawaii and *not* drink a mai tai or sample the freshest, best-tasting pineapple on the planet?

You should, if that's something that brings you joy. We all get knocked off the path at one point or another. Persistence means you can *get back* on the highway after taking a detour.

Persistence keeps us moving forward. Then when a distraction presents itself, you can do the evaluation. The Friday night drinks might be the low-value detour that isn't worth it, whereas the trip to Hawaii most definitely is.

And what about the world's largest wooden beaver? Well, that's your call.

PROGRESSION

Once you've made some lifestyle changes and stuck with them for a while, you've likely started to see some change. You're moving. If you set your cruise control, you'll keep moving, although it might not feel like it, because you've stopped accelerating. Acceleration makes driving fun— progression makes your wellness journey fun.

You've set a new baseline in strength, body measurement, or another health marker. It's time to work a little harder and accelerate. You know your car can handle it. Once you feel comfortable with the changes you've made, it might be time to turn off the cruise control and gently press down on the gas pedal.

I say *gently* because progress should be controlled and managed. I remember some advice from my driver's ed teacher, Coach Bennett. He said, "A good driver makes everyone in the car feel relaxed and safe." If you're jerky and swerving around, you risk too much.

Three years ago, I was doing CrossFit as a part of my training. It was fun to progress—to accelerate. But I let my ego get in the way and I injured my back. I wasn't a good driver that day.

Push, but stay in control. Everyone in the car (including your muscles, bones, ligaments, and tendons) should enjoy the ride and get stronger with you.

THE INEVITABLE FOURTH P: PLATEAUS

Plateaus are the villains of this story. The first three Ps help us on the road to wellness, but this fourth P is insidious because it seems to discount all of the great work we're doing. Like I said, our bodies love homeostasis. That's why everyone eventually faces a plateau.

Here's what a wellness plateau looks like: over the course of two months, you go from only being able to do one push-up at a time to being able to do ten push-ups without stopping. Each training session you feel stronger and stronger, but for the last few you haven't progressed. You're stuck at ten.

Plateaus can go on for months. If you don't recognize that they're a natural part of the process, they can defeat the other three Ps. You put in the work, training regularly and pushing hard, but you're just not getting stronger. It can be incredibly discouraging.

Plateaus will mentally drain you, especially if you've had recent success. You know what that success and progress feel like, so when they get taken away, you feel it more acutely. You feel stuck and maybe you want to quit.

You drive from Pensacola Beach to Philadelphia, and you get stuck in a beltway circling Charlotte, North Carolina. Rather than looking back and seeing how far you've already driven, you look ahead and say, "Philly is so far away."

When a client tells me they've plateaued, I first remind them how far they've come. I tell them to realize this is just a ledge on the mountain. They might not be gaining altitude, but they're still on the mountain and they need to keep pressing on.

I had a client named Nadine who had plateaued with her

back squats. She could handle the weight, but her form would break down, especially when she was into the last few reps of her final set. Instead of continuing to grind out training sessions at that weight, hoping she'd break through the plateau, we switched tactics. I had her switch to front squats.

With front squats, she had to use a lower weight than with the back squat. How did she get stronger using lower weight? Because the front squat forced her to be more upright, which helped strengthen her core, which is what I suspected was holding her back. Six weeks later, she made a new personal record on her back squat, all because we identified her limiting factor and made changes to address this weakness. She was off the ledge and climbing again.

Plateaus take patience and persistence to overcome. When you find yourself stuck, this is a good time to mix things up—try new tactics. In my opinion, as hard as they are to deal with, plateaus are great learning moments.

PERIODIZATION

Another tactic used to limit plateaus is called period-ization. With this approach, you change your training programming every six to eight weeks. By forcing these changes into your programming, you ensure your body is always dealing with newness. Plateaus are inevitable—you can never eliminate them completely. Your only recourse is to recognize them and quickly decide how you'll overcome them.

DETOURS OR HIGHWAYS?

Whether you want to lose seventy pounds, do a single pull-up after doing none for the last twenty years, or run in a 5K with your granddaughter, realize that it will take time to reach your vision. You *do* have your coordinates plugged into your GPS, but this GPS doesn't give you an exact time frame to reach your destination.

You're building a lifestyle that you can only achieve through patience, persistence, and progression. The journey takes time. If you have a detour here and there—a family event where you'll miss a few training sessions, your aunt Margaret offering you one of her homemade cookies, or one too many glasses of wine with your friends—you must have the persistence to get back on the highway as soon as possible. And we all need to get to our destination happy and healthy, so progress at a safe speed.

Your vision will keep you focused on your end goal, which makes it easier for you to drive right past the world's largest wooden beaver, white alligator farm, and your coworker's happy-hour invitation, and stay on the road to wellness.

CHAPTER 10

STRESS MANAGEMENT

It was a Tuesday morning in 2006, sometime in the North Las Vegas winter. The air was warm and the sky was a clear blue—a beautiful day. I had a traffic-free five-minute drive to work. But my stomach twisted into anxious knots. Why?

Because at nine o'clock, a team of nine lawyers was going to rummage through our offices, ready to take down anyone and everyone who was involved in the accounting fraud at our company. And nobody knew it was coming.

Except me.

As I said earlier in the book, I was an internal auditor—specifically, the vice president of internal audit and compliance—for a large, publicly traded company. Based on some allegations of fraud against the C-suite executives, I'd recently completed a secret internal investigation. The fraud allegations held up, so the company's board of directors went to an outside firm, and I served as their liaison during the formal investigation. I was the only one in the company who knew what was about to happen on that Tuesday morning.

It wasn't exactly like the movies; the lawyers were very methodical. They pulled the hard drives from all of the executives' computers and collected box after box after box of files. My coworkers' faces were painted with confusion, fear, and anger.

I stood there watching. I wasn't confused, afraid, or angry. I was stressed. I knew exactly how this had happened, but that didn't change the fundamental reality: the stress of the events leading up to this day had nearly broken me into pieces.

In order to help the lawyers get the hard drives from all the executives' computers, I needed help from someone in IT. Because I didn't know how far the fraud went, I couldn't directly tell the chief information officer (CIO) why I needed help, but I did give him the courtesy of asking if I could borrow one of his staff for the day.

"What's this about?" he asked.

"I can't tell you that, but it is a board-sanctioned project."

He nodded his understanding and said, "All right."

I always had good relationships with the IT guys. When I told the IT staff guy I needed his help, he was all for it. That was, until I told him what I needed him to do.

He'd have to go into the office of every C-suite executive, make a copy of his hard drive, and then give the original to the lawyer that was assigned to observe the process.

I added, "If anyone objects or has questions, tell them to come to my office." I knew nobody would cause us trouble, because I'd already informed them of what we were doing, why we were doing it, and the consequences for hindering the work the lawyers were there to do.

I had just asked this young man to go against every hierarchal instinct and all decorum he'd ever learned in business school. He was about to take a huge risk and betray his personal relationships in order to do what was best for the company. The look on his face said it all: just the thought of going through with this assignment made him sick to his stomach. He was already on the brink of a breakdown just as I walked him through the process.

Trust me. I know exactly how you feel.

He did exactly as instructed, and the attorneys left with

seven laptop hard drives and dozens of boxes of files. We went on to repeat this process in our offices in the UK and Spain.

After that Tuesday morning with the lawyers, the investigation went on for another four and a half months. In the end, the CEO was fired, the CFO resigned, and the rest of the C-suite left standing saw me as nothing but a traitor.

I'd like to say things were better after that, but they weren't. Life at a company that's being delisted from the New York Stock Exchange (NYSE), facing multiple class-action lawsuits, and dealing with activist shareholders is not a fun place to be. The stress was chronic, and it completely derailed my health—mentally, physically, and everything in between.

This was two years after my moment on the beach. I had been on a good path, but I suddenly gained back all the weight, and once again I was looking and feeling like a fat bastard because I wasn't sleeping properly, I wasn't eating well, and I was still in that toxic relationship. I was stressed out of my gourd, and I had no tools to help me deal with that stress.

TYPES OF STRESS

There are two kinds of stress:

- Acute stress
- Chronic stress

ACUTE STRESS

A momentary stress-inducing event causes your body to release cortisol, the fight-or-flight hormone I mentioned in earlier chapters. It's the same hormone you release when you're in the woods and a bear starts chasing after you. It triggers the survival instinct in your body, and it can be very useful in a life-and-death scenario.

We were designed to deal with acute stress. We see the thing that scares us, we act by running or fighting, and the event is over. The cortisol gives you energy to do what you must do in the moment. The action then burns off the cortisol and you go back to an unstressed state.

A bear has never chased me, but I experienced a similar acute stress when I was face-to-face with the CEO. He thought I had betrayed him and the company we both worked for. He never physically chased me, but he did threaten my financial well-being. I couldn't run or fight when we met, so my cortisol level stayed elevated longer than my body was prepared for. That's not good. It needs to be brought down sooner rather than later.

THAT SCARED THE CRAP OUT OF ME

There is a reason many people enjoy scary movies. We know we're safe in the movie theater or wrapped up in a blanket on our couch, but when the bad guy shows up on screen, cortisol pumps us up with energy. We might scream, jump, or both. It feels good in short, controlled bursts.

But when the fear is real, there's a reason we poop or pee ourselves. Beyond that energy surge, our bodies shut down the functions we don't need, to help us either escape the threat or fight back. And this goes much deeper than controlling our bowel and bladder. Many of the functions that get shut off are very important to our overall wellness.

CHRONIC STRESS

Now, what happened when the investigation went on for months and I had to deal with the CEO every day? I was in a constant high-cortisol state. That's what we call chronic stress.

My situation was extreme in that I worked for a company being actively delisted from the NYSE, but most of us are dealing with some kind of chronic stress every day. There are a lot of bears and nowhere to run. Whether it's a sick loved one, a bad relationship, a hairy lawsuit, or a daily commute in traffic that just won't move fast enough (bears shouldn't have driver's licenses), things just seem to keep coming at you.

Chronic stress undermines your other wellness efforts. Cortisol, as I've said before, is a catabolic hormone, meaning it breaks down muscle. So what happens if you train hard every day, but you're constantly stressed? You won't get the results you're looking for because you're negatively impacting your body's ability to repair itself.

Our bodies weren't designed to be in constant fight-or-flight mode. Cortisol forces our body to focus on surviving the situation at hand—even if it's unnecessary—at the expense of other processes, such as muscle building, losing body fat, or reducing cardiovascular disease risk.

For many of us, the bear is always there. So how do you deal with it?

ELIMINATION

The best course of action for chronic stress is to eliminate that stress. If your job is causing constant stress, then you may have to consider changing jobs. That's what I did, eventually. Once the company returned to stability and I felt they didn't need me in the same capacity, I found another job. The CEO was gone, but there were other people who found a way to continue making my job very stressful.

I eventually built up the gumption to break up with the toxic girlfriend, which was even more difficult than quitting my job. When your car is overheating, and the stress is too much to handle without putting your whole journey at risk, you may have to pull over and drop off a passenger who constantly takes you off your wellness path.

Eliminating stressors in your life doesn't necessarily mean you have to quit your job or end a relationship. You might be able to change roles at work. Maybe the stress you feel as a result of your relationship can be fixed through counseling. Sometimes acknowledging the stress and talking about it is enough.

Whatever course of action you take, you have the right to eliminate as much unnecessary stress from your life as possible. You are the driver. If the relationships, jobs, and other facets of your life are causing you chronic stress, you need to address them because they're preventing you from being the healthy, vibrant individual you deserve to be.

CHANGE ENVIRONMENTS

For some people, your actual environment may be enough to cause chronic stress. When I was twenty-five years old in 1991 and a master's student at Southern Miss, I passed the CPA exam. After the exam, I went to Pensacola Beach for a four-day vacation, my first as an adult.

With my toes in the sand and the sun shining down on me, I realized that this was my happy place. I'd never been there before, but the beach gave me something I didn't get elsewhere—peace.

Throughout my life, I went where the work took me (I've lived in thirteen different states). I count myself fortunate to have had that experience, but I didn't take the time to consider the whole me. Money and recognition (i.e., job title) don't buy you wellness, especially when it comes with chronic stress.

I now call Pensacola Beach home, and my stress level is lower than it has ever been. As I write this, my wife and I are considering even lower-maintenance lifestyles to further reduce stress.

I've chosen the path of least resistance. Yes, I make less money, but I'm where I want to be. I help people with their health and fitness, and I'm passionate about it, so it makes me happy.

What kind of lifestyle you want is important, but figuring out what kind of lifestyle you *need* is just as vital. Many vows include the promise to stick through "sickness and health," but your wellness vow did not. You want wellness and, in turn, happiness. Chronic stress robs you of happiness.

We believe stress is a part of daily life and we just have to accept it. You don't. In fact, chronic stress can have a direct impact on your longevity. In other words, chronic stress isn't a way of life—it's a way of death.

THREE TECHNIQUES FOR UNAVOIDABLE STRESS

I remember when I had a Datsun (yes, I'm dating myself) that needed the brakes resurfaced. I was stressed because I knew there was a point of no return where the repair cost would quadruple, but I didn't have the money to get the work done. I could neither eliminate nor leave my stressor. I had to deal with the problem.

There are some stressors that you cannot eliminate or walk away from. That's why you need techniques to help cope with the unavoidable stress in your life.

BREATHING TECHNIQUES

In 2001, I was managing a team on a big project. It had a firm due date that was fast approaching. If we were late or there was an error in the data, the company was subject to penalties in the tens of thousands of dollars, and each day that we were late would cost more and more.

On the afternoon of the day before the project was due, the data validation coordinator, Eilene, came into my office and said, "We have a huge problem! The IT lead changed the query and now all of the data is wrong. We won't make the deadline."

The stress washed over me.

Despite my desire to run and my desire to fight the problem (i.e., hit the IT lead), I took in a deep breath. And that changed everything.

I asked myself, "What is the difference between 5:00 p.m. on Friday and 7:00 a.m. on Monday, if the client wasn't going to look at the data over the weekend?" I went to the client and they agreed to an extended deadline. I bought us two and a half days to fix the problem.

A single breath gave me the clarity I needed. That was my first experience with the value of breathing.

I already mentioned the 3-4-5 breathing technique that I learned from Dr. Chatterjee: breathe in for three seconds, hold for four, and breathe out for five. It is similar to box breathing where you breathe in, hold, breathe out, and hold all for the same fixed time (such as three seconds).

Some people find holding after they breathe out uncomfortable, but with practice, you'll get used to it. Whichever breathing technique you prefer, find one to help you manage stressful moments.

You can use breathing anytime—just take a few minutes in your office, your car, the bathroom, or the elevator to bring your stress level down.

MOVEMENT

For me, lifting weights is cathartic. Lifting heavy things gets me completely present in the moment and out of my head. My thoughts aren't anywhere else; I'm totally focused on the movements of the lifts, the form, the tempo, and the muscles I'm working.

Most runners experience the same phenomenon. They get into a state where they release endorphins and their troubles seem to melt away. Whether it is lifting, running, or walking, movement is a stress reducer. How cool is that? You're improving your fitness and managing stress.

MEDITATION

Meditation might just be leaving the realm of woo-woo and entering the mainstream. In fact, if you were to interview successful people, you'd find that most of them meditate or pray. These activities help us deal with our feelings and emotions from a very different perspective. And it doesn't have to have a religious connotation either.

You can never separate yourself from your thoughts and emotions, but you can try to have a more objective view. Just as that deep breath did in the moment of a missed deadline, meditation helps you take a step back and see things differently. The only difference is that with meditation, you practice building a more resilient, present mindset. It won't make you bulletproof to stress, but it will help you sort out the bits that don't really matter in the grand scheme of things.

Meditation isn't always about sitting still in a quiet place. You can indeed find meditative moments through movement, rather than sitting cross-legged on a pillow. For me, that happens in the gym or as I walk on the beach; for you, meditation might mean walking through nature or playing music. The most important thing is finding a way to be present in the moment without letting your emotions and thoughts affect you. That takes practice.

If you are combining these three practices regularly—breathing, movement, and meditation—along with eliminating the major stressors in your life, you'll create a holistic stress-management practice that makes you more resistant to stress.

DON'T OVERHEAT

Your car's engine has a standard temperature range within which it operates. The car requires combustion to move—there will always be heat and stress on the engine. Think of these stress-reduction practices like the radiator on a car. The radiator helps the engine stay at a good operating temperature. The more you practice various stress-reduction methods, the better your radiator will work.

The techniques I've outlined in this chapter provide the radiator fluid in your engine to help dissipate some of the heat so you don't burn up. I encourage you to use them and find other activities and tools to help you let the heat escape.

But above all, don't stress about stress. I've found the best way to not stress is to seek joy. Make a point of adding joy to each day. It can be as simple as taking a walk with a friend, or journaling about the things you're grateful for, or petting your dog or cat. Joy is the ultimate antistressor.

THE STREETS CAN BE TOUGH

As we roll off the STREETS, I know I've given you a lot of food for thought. The STREETS are where we enact our strategies and tactics. The rubber hits the road and you make it happen.

It starts with strategies. Set strategies that keep you moving forward, and as you progress and take detours, use those times as learning moments to develop even better strategies. Having a good set of strategies will help you avoid most of the roadblocks and potholes life brings your way.

Your progress will require you to train to get down the road quicker. You have to work to achieve and keep the wellness you deserve. When your training is designed to get you to your vision, it becomes a part of you.

As you train harder, you need to prioritize sleep. Learn how to rest and recover.

Proper nutrition will give your body the energy, building materials, and enjoyment you need to reach your vision. Eat real food. And drink plain old water (POW).

Experiment to find the tactics that work for you. Find your big rocks, put them in your jar, and shake it.

Remember that great results take time to reach. Stay patient, be persistent, and keep progressing. You'll be amazed at how far you can go if you don't let the plateaus stop you.

Own stress rather than allowing it to own you. This was

the hardest part for me. Now that I'm actively working on lowering my stress level, my wellness is on an upward trajectory.

As you work your way through the STREETS, you'll learn so much about yourself. Build your wellness roadmap. It will be a great tool for getting to your vision and beyond.

PART 3

—

CARGO

In part 3, I want to help you celebrate your accomplishment, get comfortable with your new self, prepare for the new attention you'll receive from other people, and wrap your mind around your new, healthier self.

First of all, congratulations! You've done what the majority of people won't: you've taken major steps to improve your wellness.

I say *won't* instead of *can't* for a reason. Most people *can* make changes that would improve their happiness, health, and fitness, but they just refuse to do it. They see the big rocks, but they direct all of their attention to the grains of sand. They want the magic pill to make them well.

I recently ran a twenty-eight-day no-alcohol challenge and

posted about it on Facebook. As you might imagine, I had comments questioning my ability to do such a thing, but many of the comments were sad. People said there was no way they could make that change, not even for a few weeks, even though they knew it would improve their health.

For most of those people, their problem isn't with their body—it's with their mind. They think they can't change themselves, which in turn makes it true. You, on the other hand, have changed your mindset for the better, which puts you at the front of the pack on the road to wellness.

You've made a lot of changes to get to your vision. Some of them were small and some of them were huge. Maybe you've never exercised before, and now you're exercising regularly. Maybe you're meditating regularly, or you're journaling your sleep habits every night.

At the start, I find that most people set a low bar. They limit their vision based on where they are at the time. As they pass mile marker after mile marker, something wonderful happens—they open their eyes and see further down the road. The journey gets more enjoyable, and they reach their vision.

Setting a low bar at first is OK, because when you reach that vision, regardless of how far you've come from the start, you'll feel like a different person. You've gone through all of the obstacles on the road, you've remained focused, and now you're at your destination. You should feel different because you are different.

It's time to unload the CARGo.

If you've ever gone to a high school reunion, then I'm pretty sure you've endured the guy who can't stop talking about his perfect game way back then (maybe ladies do this, too, but it always seems to be a guy). He seems to have peaked at seventeen and hasn't done anything since. Don't be like that guy at the high school reunion. Don't rest on your accomplishments. Keep pushing forward.

You've done something special by setting your Wellness GPS. Keep your foot on that gas pedal. This is not your peak; it is simply a higher vantage point. From this point, you can see higher visions to strive for and reach, but let's take a moment to stop and smell the roses.

In 2007, I bought a Can-Am Spyder motorcycle. It was basically a crotch rocket, except with three wheels. It was much more powerful than anything I'd ever driven. The speedometer went up to 200, and while I'll neither confirm nor deny making any efforts to test that 200-mile-per-hour limit, it sure was fun to drive. Being healthier and fit is also fun, so enjoy it. That's why the C in CARGo stands for celebrate.

While the Spyder was technically a motorcycle, it didn't really operate like one. I had to learn this new ride—it turned differently, the brakes worked differently, and it handled differently. You, too, will have to get used to handling your new, fitter body.

Because the Spyder was new and didn't look like every other motorcycle, everybody stopped to look at it. They'd even go so far as to come up to me to ask about it. Being an introvert, that wasn't natural or comfortable for me. I had to adjust to how people looked at and treated me. I wasn't anonymous like I was in my pickup truck.

Similarly, you'll have to adjust to how people treat you with your new body. The *A* in CARGo stands for adjusting to your new self. You'll have to adjust to your new feelings, your new fitness, and your new lifestyle. You'll also have to adjust to how people treat you. This might seem easy, but for many people, it is not.

Once you adjust to your new normal, you will start to realize that this is not your peak physical condition. After I'd had my Spyder for a year, I set my sights on the Samson Switchblade flying car. The Switchblade hasn't hit production, and my priorities have changed, but who knows? Maybe one day. The *R* in CARGo stands for resetting your GPS.

Then it's time to Go! If you learned anything on this journey, it was that you have to shake the jar, put your foot on the gas, and act. Be the driver and get yourself to your new vision.

CELEBRATE

The vast majority of people quit before they ever reach the point you're at now. It reminds me of a story about a gold miner from the 1840s. He bought a gold mine in California, hoping to cash in on the gold rush. He dug in that mine for months and never struck gold. Defeated, he gave up and sold the mine for pennies on the dollar.

The man who bought the mine discovered something incredible once he started digging himself: the previous owner had stopped three feet short of a massive vein of gold worth a fortune.

Most people are like that first prospector: they get within feet of the gold without realizing it, then, forgetting how far they've come, they walk away. They wanted to lose thirty-five pounds, and with a restrictive diet and daily killer bouts on the treadmill, they lost *only* twenty-five pounds. Without patience or persistence, they failed to continue educating themselves about better tactics, such as better sleep and stress reduction, that might have given them that final push.

But you did make the final push, and you've made this phenomenal change. You should celebrate that fact.

In the United States, most of our celebrations center on food, and that's a great thing. But what foods do we associate with each holiday? Birthdays mean cake, Thanksgiving means stuffing and gravy and pies, the Fourth of July means hot dogs and beer, and Halloween means candy. Those foods are ingrained in the specific celebration, and almost all of them are terrible for you.

The celebration for you reaching your initial vision should be in line with that vision, not against it. Don't let an unhealthy spread at the celebration send you back toward your starting point.

For me, the Tough Mudder race with Bekah was both part of my vision and my celebration. Just before the finish line, there was an obstacle that required us to run through a series of live electric wires. My daughter and I rounded the corner and saw a group of men in their twenties and thirties staring at the wires with trepidation. They'd seen others run into one of those wires, fall into the ground face-first, and immediately try to get up, only to get knocked down by another wire.

I told my daughter to run around them. I grasped her hand and we charged into the obstacle. Yes, we both got shocked, and, yes, I almost fell over, but we both kept moving forward. We came out the other side and finished the race together. It was everything I'd worked toward. Pure joy. That was my celebration.

Your celebration might take a different form than being electrocuted with your child, but whatever it is, it has to reinforce that you've accomplished something incredible with your wellness, and you're going to accomplish even more.

Gorging yourself on cake doesn't quite get the job done.

ADJUSTING TO YOUR NEW NORMAL

You are a different person. You should expect to feel different and be treated differently.

HOW YOU SEE YOURSELF

My client Trent has used much of the advice I've given you throughout this book, and he has gotten great results. He's a regular at the gym, and he's become comfortable around all the twenty-year-olds.

Recently, Trent sent me an email with an attachment. It was a picture of a shirtless Trent with a big smile on his face. He looked great!

He's out of his comfort zone now. Don't mistake this for a garden variety of vanity. When vanity comes unearned, it is typically associated with how someone looks relative to other people. *Earned* vanity comes from comparing yourself to who you used to be. Earned vanity is good for us because it is tied to the work we've done. Trent had earned his vanity.

If you don't like the word *vanity*, call it feeling sexy. You have every right to feel sexy now.

One of my first clients was a fifty-three-year-old Marine named Sandra. She'd had a heart attack and had gotten incredibly unfit since leaving the military. In her words, she hated exercise—even when she was in the service, she'd hated the physical training.

With her, I took a different approach than with most of my clients: I focused on food choices more than anything else and made sure her training was more focused on play. I encouraged her to play with her granddaughter, which turned out to be good exercise even though she didn't think of it as training.

About two months into her training with me, she had already surpassed anything she thought she was capable of, including losing fifteen pounds off her five-foot-three-inch frame. The changes she was making were already having an incredible effect on her body measurements, too. In fact, Sandra's granddaughter even made a comment about her grandma's new body: "When I get big, I want to have strong arms just like Grandma."

I thought the comment was awesome, and I figured it would motivate Sandra even more, but it actually had the opposite effect for her. She couldn't handle the extra attention.

As a result, she stopped training with me.

Sandra's response seems strange to a lot of people, but I came to understand why: humans are creatures of habit. We like patterns for our behavior. We get used to people treating us a certain way and only paying attention to us in a certain way, so once people respond to us differently than we're used to, it interrupts the pattern of how we see ourselves. It can be incredibly disconcerting, and it can be enough to make some people stop their journey.

As a part of unloading the CARGo from your car after a long journey, you must get comfortable with your new reality. You have a new lifestyle and people will ask you questions about your progress. It might seem invasive, or it might seem flattering. Just keep your mind focused on your *why* and your vision. The GPS is telling you that you've reached your destination. Adjust to your new environment and enjoy the view.

HOW OTHER PEOPLE SEE YOU

Of course you can see that you're different—you see it in the mirror and you see it in how your clothes fit (if you're even wearing the same clothes). But other people will also see you differently now. Go ahead and share your journey with them, but don't expect their excitement to last. You've done what very few people have ever done: you dug the extra three feet. In your mind, you know you had to dig, but all they'll see is the gold you discovered.

They'll want to know all the shortcuts you took—the magic pill. All I can suggest is that you hand them this book.

They can't use your roadmap because, like I've said, it's different for everybody. You can tell them you did keto, and they'll say they could never eat like that. You'll say you did HIIT, and they'll say they don't have time to run. Some people will pooh-pooh everything. Don't feel compelled to save them. You can hand them this framework to create their roadmap and let them set their own GPS, but it's up to them to drive. They have to get behind the steering wheel and drive themselves. You can only open the driver's side door and encourage them to start.

CRABS IN A BUCKET

I spoke of saboteurs in chapter 3, Self-Awareness. They'll still be around at this point in your journey. In fact, new ones might even surface. You might hear, "You're getting too skinny!" Before you let them get into your head, take a look at where they're getting their idea of "skinny." With the current obesity rate, a normal body type does look skinny by comparison. Take what they're saying as well-meaning, but don't let it affect your new lifestyle.

It is the *evil* saboteurs who will sound off the loudest.

I remember, as a teenager, going crabbing in Manchac, Louisiana. My parents would take traps out with the boat, and the *kids* would crab from the dock. We'd use a string, a turkey neck, a net, and a ton of patience.

We'd tie one end of the string to the turkey neck and toss the neck into the water. After a few minutes, we slowly brought the turkey neck up to the surface. Often, a crab would be gnawing on the turkey. We got them as close to the surface as we could and then scooped them up with the net. We then tossed them in the bucket and kept going.

After a good day, the bucket would be almost full. Although many of the crabs were near the top, they seldom got out, because all of the other crabs pulled them back down. That's how evil saboteurs work—they want to pull others down to get on top.

But you've gotten out of the bucket, and you can leave the other crabs (evil saboteurs) in that bucket.

IS A LOWER METABOLISM A PROBLEM?

Some people will wonder if you starved yourself to get to where you are. They'll say you dieted and that's not sustainable, because you lowered your metabolism and that's bad for you. However, there's solid science showing that a lower metabolism actually leads to a longer life.[11]

Yes, *The Biggest Loser* contestants did lower their metabolism, and that's part of the reason why they put on weight after the show, but they also put on weight because they didn't change their habits—they didn't use the wellness roadmap to build a sustainable lifestyle. So don't worry about lowering your metabolism because you watched your nutrition—a lower metabolism can actually be good for you.

Your body has found a new homeostasis, and if you're able to thrive at this new place, that's a good thing.

It is worth repeating: if people treat you negatively at this point in your journey, they're only responding to how they feel about themselves. It's not about you—it's about them.

---

11   Jonathan Shaw, "A New Theory on Longevity," *Harvard Magazine*, November–December 2004, https://harvardmagazine.com/2004/11/a-new-theory-on-longevit.html.

Don't let the fact that some crabs try to pull you down keep you from enjoying your success.

You don't have to worry about those crabs who hold you back because, you've met some other escapees along the road to wellness (your accountability team).

NEW FRIENDS

More important than the haters are the new friends you made on your journey. You'll have accountability partners who support you and want to learn from your methods. You'll also have old friends you haven't seen in years commending you on how amazing you look and wanting to start their own wellness journey.

The good news is that you're around more people who are like-minded—focused on health and fitness—and they'll understand the importance and difficulty of what you've accomplished so far. They'll be the community of people who support you as you drive forward.

TAKEAWAY

You've probably heard the saying that success is a journey, not a destination. The roadmap helps you get to a specific spot, but it's more of a waypoint than a final destination. You still have so much in front of you. You've reached only your initial vision. You have so many more possibilities now that you've proven to yourself what you're capable of. How will you move forward to the next destination on your wellness journey?

RESETTING YOUR GPS

I've seen people get stuck at this point more times than I can count. They reach their initial vision, and then they fail to reset their GPS, so they meander around until their engine sputters and they lose ground. Maintenance is great, but remember how much fun acceleration was?

Trent is the perfect example of someone who did not meander and took a great interest in building on what he'd already accomplished. Trent wanted to lose weight, which he did; then he wanted to put on muscle, which he is doing.

So many people get comfortable being unhealthy. A funk settles over them, and in an odd way, they get comfortable in the funk. Most people accept their unhealthy lives, especially as they get older and don't know anything else. However, you've climbed a mountain, and from this vantage point, you can see that you can climb to an even higher peak. You can do so much more.

You can choose to maintain, do more, or regress. I will tell you right now, doing nothing is a sure way to regress.

Revisit the GPS from the beginning. You don't have to redo everything in terms of grounding and gaining self-awareness, because you likely have a better sense of those factors now. But you do want to use the GPS chapters as a platform to see where you need to go next.

Revisit the reason why you started this journey to begin with. Has your *why* changed since the first go-round? It might be more specific or more personal. My *why* changed a bit because I married Tammy six months after I reached my first vision. Use this time to deeply connect or reconnect with your *why*.

You're stronger now, so maybe you want to join a gym and start lifting free weights. Or maybe with your improved mobility and balance you're ready to learn a martial art or join a tennis club. You might have built the endurance to keep up with your grandchildren and you'd like to coach their soccer team to spend more time with them. This is the time to reach for a higher vision.

It might be a place you've never been and it might scare you a bit. That's a good thing.

Some couples renew their vows after their five-year or ten-year anniversary. With your updated *why* and vision, you might have to renew your vow to yourself.

Make this commitment of self-love for the next phase of your journey.

Now you can personalize this by reevaluating your baselines and setting new SMART goals (mile markers). Your baselines have likely changed—your body measurements and health markers probably look better than when you first started. Maybe you brought your blood sugar down slightly and you want to get it to a point where you don't need medication at all. Now might be the time to push further on your nutrition and see if you can get your A1C and fasting glucose numbers down.

Maybe you want to get your endurance up so you can go cross-country skiing with your kids and grandkids. Or like me, you can look for ways to eliminate chronic stress so you can have more joy in your life. Measure the baseline and set the first SMART mile marker toward that vision.

As for self-awareness, you probably have a pretty good grasp of who you are now. But there is one thing to be aware of this time. Be ready for a potentially slower progression than when you set your GPS the first time. Don't worry, that's normal.

You might have seen incredible results at the beginning of your wellness journey. You did twice as many push-ups in week two than in week one, you ran twice as far, or you walked twice as many blocks. Understand that you might not make that level of progress as quickly now. You've already put the big rocks in place for the most part. Now you're working with small rocks and sand. That can mean smaller and slower changes, but they're still very important.

Of course, we all have physical limitations, but you can accomplish anything and everything you set your mind to if you're willing to put in the effort to make it happen.

GO

Now that you've reset your GPS, you don't just sit there waiting for the car to take you there (autonomous cars are coming but not for the wellness journey). You have to get behind the wheel. You have to push the gas pedal and steer yourself onto the highway.

You have developed an amazing user's manual for yourself. You have a good idea of the things you need to do and how your body should respond. You know that when you properly line up your actions with your vision, you keep yourself on the road and you can see the mile markers getting closer as you go.

This time, it will be easier to know the appropriate mode of transportation to get yourself to your destination at the right pace. For you, training for a specific event such as a race allows you to get in the fast lane with a sports car. Or you may still have passengers and cargo to manage. Either way, this should all be much more apparent to you this time around.

Wellness starts with a mindset shift. If you don't have the right mindset, you'll never develop the habits and lifestyle to get to your destination. Most people want to start with the tactics because they don't understand that wellness is not a destination. It is a series of destinations that we work to get to throughout our lives.

Today, you might be focused on improving your fitness, but tomorrow, you might be dealing with a chronic illness. Our journey should always lead to the most joy and the best health and fitness we can achieve for ourselves. If we're not moving forward toward wellness, we're moving away from it. That's the reality of aging.

You may feel good in your new wellness destination. It is cozy and comfortable—it would be easy to stay here. But I think you know, deep down, that there's more out there for you to see and do.

It's time to turn the key in the ignition, check the gauges, press the gas pedal, and go. The power is in your hands. The steering wheel is in your grip; your foot is on the pedal. All right, let's go!

CONCLUSION

As you progress toward even bigger visions, keep on refining your wellness roadmap by learning and experimenting. Read blogs and books and listen to podcasts to keep finding the next biggest rock. Put that rock in the jar and shake it.

Seek out opportunities to educate yourself and learn different approaches. Some of them will work very well for you, and others will have to be discarded.

Seek out people who can help you along your way. You'll gain quite a bit if you open yourself up to the perspective and guidance of experts—the people who've been there and done that—and learn from their wins and mistakes.

And above all, don't be afraid to make an investment in yourself. Wellness pays dividends well above anything else you could spend money on. The cost of being unwell, particularly when you know it is self-inflicted, should be a nonstarter for you. Invest by buying high-quality real food. Invest by buying the equipment or a gym membership that is going to help you keep your muscles and bones strong. Invest by hiring a good coach to push you and keep you on track.

If you're truly committed to change, you have to change yourself first. You could look at that as a scary proposition, but, to me, that's the most empowering advice a person can ever hear. You're in control of your destiny, and you have the power to get behind the steering wheel and take yourself where you want to go.

LET'S STAY IN TOUCH

Thank you for letting me be a part of your wellness journey. I'd love to keep the conversation going, whether that means listening to the *40+ Fitness Podcast*, letting me know how your journey is coming along, or being part of one of my coaching programs. Feel free to reach out to me. You can go to 40plusfitnesspodcast.com, where you can find past podcast episodes, information on my coaching programs, and various ways to contact me. You can also go to wellnessroadmapbook.com to learn more about programs and future books in the Wellness Roadmap series.

ACKNOWLEDGMENTS

I would like to thank the people who helped me get this book published. Greg Larson, Kate Rallis, Kayla Sokol, and the rest of the great folks at Scribe Media, you were so helpful throughout this process.

Thank you to all of the experts and authors who have been guests on the *40+ Fitness Podcast* over the past two and a half years. It is through your generous sharing of knowledge that I have been able to write this book.

And finally, I'd like to say thank you to my clients and podcast listeners. You make learning and teaching wellness the best job a man could have.

ABOUT THE AUTHOR

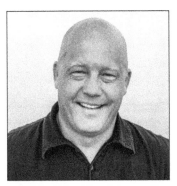

ALLAN MISNER is a National Academy of Sports Medicine (NASM) Certified Personal Trainer and a Functional Aging Institute (FAI) Certified Functional Aging Specialist. Allan is creator of the thriving 40+ Fitness Community, providing one-on-one and group fitness coaching, nutritional guidance, and personal training for clients over the age of forty. He is also the host of the *40+ Fitness Podcast*, for which he has interviewed hundreds of health and wellness experts with a wide range of specialties.